D0303939

The social psychology of food

Applying social psychology
Series editor: Stephen Sutton

Published and forthcoming titles

The social psychology of food

Mark Conner and Christopher J. Armitage

Open University Press
Buckingham · Philadelphia

Open University Press
Celtic Court
22 Ballmoor
Buckingham
MK18 1XW

email: enquiries@openup.co.uk
world wide web: www.openup.co.uk

and
325 Chestnut Street
Philadelphia, PA 19106, USA

First Published 2002

Copyright © Mark Conner and Christopher J. Armitage 2002

All rights reserved. Except for the quotation of short passages for the purpose of criticism and review, no part of this publication may be reproduced, stored in a retrieval system, or transmitted, in any form or by any means, electronic, mechanical, photocopying, recording or otherwise, without the prior written permission of the publisher or a licence from the Copyright Licensing Agency Limited. Details of such licences (for reprographic reproduction) may be obtained from the Copyright Licensing Agency Ltd of 90 Tottenham Court Road, London, W1P 0LP.

A catalogue record of this book is available from the British Library

ISBN   0 335 20754 5 (pb)   0 335 20755 3 (hb)

Library of Congress Cataloging-in-Publication Data
Conner, Mark, 1962-
  The social psychology of food / Mark Conner and Christopher J. Armitage.
    p. cm. – (Applying social psychology)
  Includes bibliographical references and index.
  ISBN 0-335-20755-3 – ISBN 0-335-20754-5 (pbk.)
    1. Food habits–Social aspects. 2. Food habits–Psychological aspects. I. Armitage, Christopher J., 1973– II. Title. III. Series.

GT2860 .C58 2002
394.1'2–dc21   2002023851

Typeset by Graphicraft Limited, Hong Kong
Printed in Great Britain by Biddles Limited, Guildford and King's Lynn

The social psychology of food

Mark Conner and Christopher J. Armitage

Open University Press
Buckingham · Philadelphia

Open University Press
Celtic Court
22 Ballmoor
Buckingham
MK18 1XW

email: enquiries@openup.co.uk
world wide web: www.openup.co.uk

and
325 Chestnut Street
Philadelphia, PA 19106, USA

First Published 2002

Copyright © Mark Conner and Christopher J. Armitage 2002

All rights reserved. Except for the quotation of short passages for the purpose of criticism and review, no part of this publication may be reproduced, stored in a retrieval system, or transmitted, in any form or by any means, electronic, mechanical, photocopying, recording or otherwise, without the prior written permission of the publisher or a licence from the Copyright Licensing Agency Limited. Details of such licences (for reprographic reproduction) may be obtained from the Copyright Licensing Agency Ltd of 90 Tottenham Court Road, London, W1P 0LP.

A catalogue record of this book is available from the British Library

ISBN   0 335 20754 5 (pb)   0 335 20755 3 (hb)

Library of Congress Cataloging-in-Publication Data
Conner, Mark, 1962-
   The social psychology of food / Mark Conner and Christopher J. Armitage.
      p. cm. – (Applying social psychology)
   Includes bibliographical references and index.
   ISBN 0-335-20755-3 – ISBN 0-335-20754-5 (pbk.)
   1. Food habits–Social aspects. 2. Food habits–Psychological aspects. I. Armitage, Christopher J., 1973– II. Title. III. Series.

GT2860 .C58 2002
394.1'2–dc21   2002023851

Typeset by Graphicraft Limited, Hong Kong
Printed in Great Britain by Biddles Limited, Guildford and King's Lynn

Contents

Series editor's foreword

Social psychology is sometimes criticized for not being sufficiently 'relevant' to everyday life. The Applying Social Psychology series challenges this criticism. It is organized around applied topics rather than theoretical issues, and is designed to complement the highly successful Mapping Social Psychology series edited by Tony Manstead. Social psychologists, and others who take a social-psychological perspective, have conducted research on a wide range of interesting and important applied topics such as consumer behaviour, work, politics, the media, crime and environmental issues. Each book in the new series takes a different applied topic and reviews relevant social-psychological ideas and research. The books are texts rather than research monographs. They are pitched at final year undergraduate level, but will also be suitable for students on Masters level courses as well as researchers and practitioners working in the relevant fields. Although the series has an applied emphasis, theoretical issues are not neglected. Indeed, the series aims to demonstrate that theory-based applications of social psychology can contribute to our understanding of important applied topics.

The Social Psychology of Food is the third book in the series. The authors are leading researchers in the field and are well known for their work applying social cognition models to food choice and dietary change. As they point out, food is central to the lives of all of us and is much more than mere sustenance. The amount, frequency and type of food that we eat are influenced by many different factors. Consider a person who goes to his works canteen for lunch. What determines his choice of meal and the quantity he consumes? Availablility and price no doubt play a role, but how important are the appearance, smell, taste and texture of the food on offer? Is he likely to choose different foods depending on his mood or how stressed he feels? To what extent will his choice be influenced by what he believes about the fat content of the food and the effect of consuming fatty foods on his risk of developing heart disease? Will he tend to eat more, or choose different items, if he is joined by his workmates rather than eating alone? These questions illustrate some of the numerous social-psychological influences on eating and food choice that are analysed by Conner and Armitage. It is only relatively recently that social psychologists have started to apply their theories and methods to understanding food-related behaviours. This book provides a lucid review of what has been learned to date on this fascinating topic and suggests several promising avenues for future research.

Stephen Sutton

Preface

Food is central to the lives of all, and has for centuries been celebrated in art, poetry and song (e.g. Smith 1996). More recently, increased concentration from the media has focused public attention on the food we eat, and its influence on physical health and mental well-being. Until relatively recently, however, food had received no more than sporadic attention from social scientists. The past couple of decades have seen significant attention paid to the important topic of food by all kinds of social scientists, and particularly those from a social psychology background. Thus, food now appears to be of considerable interest to both social scientists and members of the public. There is also now a significant body of literature on food from a social psychological perspective, and it would seem timely to publish a text reviewing this literature.

This book reviews the key current research on food from the perspective of two social psychologists. Rather than trying to be comprehensive in this coverage, we have attempted to provide a more focused coverage of particular material. In selecting what to focus on we have tried to be led by what we believe to be the important areas of current research on food. But this selection has undoubtedly also been influenced by our own biases and interests. Probably this is most obvious in relation to the methodologies of the research we review. Our own research interests tend to focus upon quantitative research methods rather than qualitative methods, and this bias is reflected in our coverage of research. However, we would not want this to be taken as indicating that we do not see the value in qualitative research; indeed, we believe that some of the best research combines both qualitative and quantitative approaches. It is also true that in reviewing material we have not restricted ourselves to purely social psychological research. Instead, we have tried to present a range of material within a particular area in order to emphasize the contribution of social psychological studies to furthering understanding. We have also shown a bias towards reporting the results of our own research where it seemed appropriate. The justification has more to do with us having the clearest grasp of this material than with any negative views on the work of others in these areas.

The chapters have been written to be self-contained and readable independently of one another. This is particularly true for Chapters 2 to 6. The first chapter provides some important background information to the approach we have taken in writing the book, and presents an overview of the rest of the book. The final chapter tries to draw together themes for further research in this area, but probably requires a good understanding of issues in the rest of the book to be of most value.

Finally, we would like to thank Sarah Grogan, Maddy Arden and Daryl O'Connor for generally being helpful and supportive during the preparation of this book and for reading and commenting upon drafts of different chapters. We would also like to thank the series editor, Steve Sutton, for his useful feedback on the book and encouraging comments. Our final thanks go to all at Open University Press for all their help and encouragement and to Justin Vaughan and Miriam Selwyn in particular.

Acknowledgements

The data in Table 3.1 were adapted from National Food Survey Branch, UK Ministry of Agriculture, Fisheries and Food. Figure 4.1 is redrawn from Bagozzi and Edwards (2000) with permission. Figure 6.1 is adapted from Lewis and Hill (1998). Table 4.1 is taken from Metropolitan Life Insurance Company tables (1983) with permission. The data in Table 4.2 are taken from Gallagher *et al.* (2000) with permission.

1

Introduction

General overview

Food plays an important part in all our lives in a variety of ways. At the lowest level of abstraction, food and drink are necessary to sustain life. However, for the vast majority of people, food is more than mere sustenance; interaction with food is pleasurable, and sometimes a source of relief from daily stress. The intake of food (consumption) also structures our daily lives, while our choice of food has implications for our waistline and our health, and even offers a way of presenting ourselves to others. Furthering our understanding of these issues is the focus of *The Social Psychology of Food*. There are a number of excellent texts that deal with the physiology of food (e.g. Capaldi 1996) and even the psychology of food (e.g. Logue 1991), but the focus here is upon what research from a *social psychological* perspective has contributed to our understanding of food-related behaviours.

This introductory chapter first provides an outline of the scope of the social psychology of food. This includes a consideration of the scope of social psychology, the methods it employs and the types of food-related behaviours they apply to. We then present a broad model of **food choice** and preference in order to place social psychological influences in a broader context of other influences. Finally, we overview the remainder of the book. Thus this introductory chapter is intended to 'set the scene' for the more detailed coverage given to topics presented in subsequent chapters.

The social psychology of food

Social psychology has been defined as the 'investigation of how the thoughts, feelings and behaviors of individuals are influenced by the actual, imagined or implied presence of others' (Allport 1935: 799). This definition places the emphasis on the importance of others in understanding our thoughts, feelings and behaviours. Nevertheless, it is assumed that this impact of others can take a variety of forms, and so the scope of social psychology extends to the vast majority of human behaviours and their thoughts and feelings about those behaviours. Social psychologists tend to be interested almost exclusively in human behaviour, and unlike a number of other areas of psychology relatively rarely use animal studies. The focus tends to be upon behaviour of various sorts (e.g. reactions of disgust to particular food; what people say), although behaviour (e.g. a smile; how people describe their feelings) is often used to infer feelings, thoughts, beliefs, attitudes, intentions and goals. What makes social psychology *social* is the idea that the subject matter deals with how people are affected by others, whether they are directly present or not.

Social cognition is an important approach within social psychology and is concerned with how individuals make sense of social situations. The approach focuses on individual cognitions or thoughts as processes that intervene between observable stimuli and responses in specific real world situations (Fiske and Taylor 1991). So, for example, social cognition approaches to understanding food choice would focus on the cognitions that intervene between perceiving a food and choosing or not choosing to consume it. Much social psychology over the past quarter-century has started from this assumption that social behaviour is best understood as a function of people's perceptions of reality, rather than as a function of the objective description of the stimulus environment. The question of which cognitions are important in predicting behaviour has been the focus of a great deal of research. This 'social cognitive' approach to the person as a thinking organism interacting with his her environment has become dominant in much of social psychology in recent years (Schneider 1991).

The *social psychology of food* is the application of the principles of social psychology to the understanding of food-related behaviours. As we have already noted, food represents far more than mere sustenance to most of us. Thus the social psychology of food is concerned with how thoughts, feelings, and behaviour impact on food choice. More broadly, it is interested in how our interaction with others and our social environment can influence what foods we eat and the amounts we eat. This has been a particularly important topic, and a broad range of disciplines have made contributions. However, while a broad range of material is presented here, the social cognition approach will be particularly dominant, because of its dominance in recent years. Rather than merely presenting the social psychological research within a particular area of food research, we have tried to provide a context by presenting a broader overview of material within that area. We hope that this manner of presenting material provides both a broader overview of material and better insights into the particular contribution of social psychological approaches.

Much of the work in social cognition can broadly be split into how people make sense of others (person **perception**) and themselves (self-regulation) (Fiske and Taylor 1991: 14). The social psychology of food is interested in how the food others eat can be used as a means of perceiving and understanding them. Food choices can also be used as a means of self-presentation. These are topics that are explored in Chapter 6. The social psychology of food is also interested in how food plays a role in our understanding of ourselves or how we regulate our own behaviour. Self-regulation processes can be defined as those 'mental and behavioral processes by which people enact their self-conceptions, revise their behavior, or alter the environment so as to bring about outcomes in it in line with their self-perceptions and personal goals' (Fiske and Taylor 1991: 181). As such, self-regulation can be seen as emerging from a clinical tradition in psychology that sees the individual as involved in behaviour change efforts designed to eliminate dysfunctional patterns of thinking or behaviour (Bandura 1982; Turk and Salovey 1986). Models of the cognitive determinants of food choice can be seen as part of this tradition. Food choice is a topic given detailed coverage in Chapter 2. Self-regulation involves the setting of goals, cognitive preparations and the ongoing monitoring and evaluation of goal-directed activities. Two phases are commonly distinguished: motivational and **volitional** (Gollwitzer 1990). The motivational phase involves deliberation on incentives and expectations in order to choose between goals and implied actions. This stage ends with a decision concerning the goal to be pursued. The second, volitional phase involves planning and action towards achieving the set goal (Conner and Norman 1996). Both these stages are important in the process of dietary change, a topic given particular attention in Chapter 3. Chapter 4 extends this research to examine an important goal in relation to the social psychology of food, that of weight control. In Chapter 5 we examine yet another influence on eating behaviour that has interested those using social psychological approaches: the impact of stress on eating. Clearly this is not an exhaustive list of topics under the heading 'the social psychology of food'. Nevertheless, these represent areas in which the contribution of social psychological approaches has been substantive.

Research methods in social psychology

A broad range of methods are used in social psychology to gain insights into social behaviours (see Manstead and Semin 1996 for detailed coverage of methods in social psychology). This range is reflected in social psychological approaches to food. Nevertheless, these methods can be broadly grouped into experimental and correlational methods.

Experimental methods are characterized by an examination of the relationship between one or more manipulated (independent) variables and a dependent variable. All other influences are held constant or controlled. Thus some studies have used experimental methods under laboratory conditions to control the effect of extraneous influences (i.e. the laboratory experiment). In order to control other factors participants are randomly allocated to experimental and control groups. The experimental group receives the manipulation that changes the independent variable, while the control group receives no manipulation. The random allocation to groups is intended to ensure that any differences between participants are averaged across groups and so have no major impact on the results. For example, Chaiken and Pliner (1987) used experimental methods to look at the impact of gender and meal size on perceptions of the target individual (see Chapter 6). They randomly allocated individuals to read 'diaries' where the diarist ate either large or small meals and was either male or female (i.e. four conditions in a 2×2 design). The dependent variables measured were perceived femininity, masculinity, concern with appearance and attractiveness. A significant impact of gender or meal size on such perceptions was indicated by significant differences in the dependent variables across conditions. Other studies eschew the laboratory and carry out experiments in real world settings (with similar assessment of the relationship between a manipulated independent variable and an observed dependent variable), but do not randomly allocate participants to conditions (i.e. a field experiment). For example, Redd and de Castro (1992), examining the impact of the presence of others on the amount eaten, instructed individuals to eat normally, eat alone or eat with others for the next five days (see Chapter 6). Self-reported amount eaten was the key dependent variable.

Another commonly used method in social psychological research on food is the correlational method. Here the focus of interest is on the relationship between two or more variables, usually in real world settings. Instead of one variable being manipulated and the effect on another observed, the variables are measured in a sample of individuals and the relationship between the two is assessed (e.g. by correlation). For example, Conner *et al.* (1999) were interested in the impact of daily stressors on the consumption of snack foods (see Chapter 5). In their study they assessed both the number of stressors individuals reported experiencing and the number of snacks they reported consuming. The relationship between the two was assessed by calculating the correlation between the two. A positive correlation significantly greater than zero was obeserved, indicating that as the number of stressors increased, so did the number of snacks eaten.

Two key considerations in the evaluation of research methods are reliability and validity. The experimental and correlational methods have a number of complementary characteristics in relation to aspects of reliability and validity. For example, laboratory experiments tend to be high in internal validity (i.e. they provide strong evidence of causal relationships between independent and dependent variables) but more suspect in relation to external validity (i.e. they do not provide good evidence of relationships that will necessarily apply in real world situations). In contrast, correlational methods tend to be considered to have good external validity but weak internal validity. The weakness of correlational methods in relation to internal validity is because observing a correlation between two variables does not imply that the first variable caused the second. It may be that the direction of causation is reversed or that a third variable caused the correlation between the first two variables. The power of correlational methods in relation to external validity can take a variety of forms. Temporal validity concerns the extent to which the findings can be replicated at different time points. Ecological validity is concerned with the extent to which the findings can be replicated in different samples or in different locations. Where different methods point to similar explanations we can be most confident in the research findings. However, such triangulation of findings across methods is not always possible. Indeed, variations in findings between studies and between methodologies may suggest new questions for research.

The above methods can all be grouped under the heading of 'scientific methods'. This approach tends to focus on the testing and refuting of hypotheses based on quantitative data. These tests are usually based upon various statistical methods (Howell 1992). Other approaches focus more on qualitative approaches to understanding, and do not necessarily draw upon scientific principles. These approaches are only now beginning to be widely applied within the social psychology of food and are therefore not a particular focus for this book. Readers interested in these approaches and their contribution to understanding food-related behaviour should consult Smith (2002).

Now that we have briefly introduced the scope and methods of the social psychology of food, the next section in this chapter considers the range of influences on food choice and the place of social psychological influences within this range. The topic is then given further, in-depth, coverage in Chapter 2.

General models of the factors influencing food choice and food preferences

Several different models of the influences upon food choice have been proposed. Early attempts (e.g. Yudkin 1956) split the factors influencing food choice into three categories: physical factors included geography, season, economics and food technology; social factors included religion, social class, nutrition education and advertising; and physiological factors included heredity, allergy, therapeutic diets, acceptability and nutritional needs. More recent conceptions (e.g. Randall and Sanjur 1981; Booth and Shepherd 1988; Shepherd 1989) generally split the influences into those factors related to the food, to the individual and to the environment. A distillation of these differing representations of the influences upon food choices is given in Figure 1.1. External factors linked to the food and the environment are assumed to influence sensory, psychological and physiological factors within the individual, and together these produce food acceptance or rejection behaviour in terms of food choices and food intake. A particular focus of this book is on the social psychological variables (under the heading 'psychological variables' in Figure 1.1).

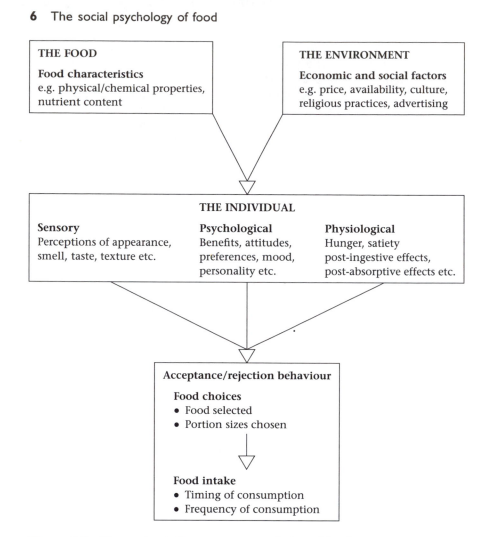

THE FOOD

Food characteristics
e.g. physical/chemical properties,
nutrient content

THE ENVIRONMENT

Economic and social factors
e.g. price, availability, culture,
religious practices, advertising

THE INDIVIDUAL

Sensory
Perceptions of appearance,
smell, taste, texture etc.

Psychological
Benefits, attitudes,
preferences, mood,
personality etc.

Physiological
Hunger, satiety
post-ingestive effects,
post-absorptive effects etc.

Acceptance/rejection behaviour

Food choices
• Food selected
• Portion sizes chosen

Food intake
• Timing of consumption
• Frequency of consumption

Figure 1.1 The major influences on our choice of food

The food

The first set of influences upon food choice can be linked to the physical composition of the food. The physical composition of the food will have effects on food choice through three routes within the individual (Figure 1.1): via sensory attributes of the food, via physiological effects of the food and via psychological effects of the food. Aspects of the food, such as its chemical and physical composition, give rise to properties of the food, which are perceived by the individual as sensory characteristics such as appearance, taste and smell. It is not the sensory characteristics themselves that lead to food choices and food intake, but preferences for particular combinations of characteristics in different eating contexts. This is because there are very few common features of foods that are universally palatable or unpalatable. Instead, the acceptability of a sensory attribute such as bitterness will be learnt by the individual through exposure to foods. Thus we learn that a particular level of sweetness in a cup of coffee is acceptable and other levels are not (Conner 1991). While it is true that there may be agreement between individuals within the same culture on the appropriate attributes of particular foods (e.g. coffee should be bitter, but ice cream should be sweet) and even agreement on the most preferred level of an attribute (e.g. how sweet people like lemonade to be). It is also true that there are large differences between people in their liking of particular foods and for levels of an attribute within a food.

In addition to producing sensory effects, the chemical composition of the food includes nutrients such as protein, carbohydrates, fat, minerals and vitamins that are vital to the functioning of the organism. Indeed, many theories of food choice emphasize the life-sustaining aspect of food ingestion over all others. Ingestion of the chemicals in foods may have other physiological effects. For instance, the consumption of high-energy food will lead to satiation and the reduction of subsequent food consumption (Blundell and Rogers 1991). Similarly, if the food leads to vomiting and sickness the food will probably be avoided in the future (Rozin and Vollmecke 1986). Thus the chemical or physical properties of the food have an influence on subsequent food choice and intake through post-ingestional effects. Individuals learn these effects and base subsequent food choices upon easily recognizable characteristics of the food which have become linked to these effects (Booth 1985).

The third way in which the chemical and physical properties of the food will affect food choice and intake is through the post-ingestional effects of consuming particular foods on psychological functioning. For example, some foods affect mood or sleepiness and it is possible that association between these effects and a particular food might influence subsequent selection of the food under appropriate circumstances.

The environment

A second set of external factors that influence food choice (Figure 1.1) are the general social and cultural environment (Rozin 1990). Food choices differ between cultures, and the social milieu surrounding individuals will impact on their food choices. Religion, for instance, may require that certain dietary choices are made regardless of personal preferences. The availability of food, its price and aspects of advertising and marketing will all have a further influence on individual food choices.

The individual

In addition to the external influences on food choices there are also influences located within the individual (Figure 1.1). As already noted, these include physiological factors, psychological factors and sensory factors that are likely to interact with aspects of the food and the environment to produce food choice. Physiological factors within the individual likely to influence food choice include hormone levels, illness, intolerance to particular food constituents and a range of other factors. Psychological differences between individuals also affect food choices. Factors such as personality have been shown to influence food choices. Part of this effect may be through different lifestyles adopted by individuals with differing personalities (Turner 1979). In a similar way, differing levels of education and nutritional knowledge will lead to different food use. Differences between individuals in previous experiences and learning associated with foods will lead to differences in beliefs, values and **habits** concerning particular foods. Furthermore, for particular occasions, different foods will be seen to be more or less appropriate. **Attitudes** of individuals towards the consumption of differing foods also constitute a major determinant of many food choices. Such attitudes are likely to be based upon a range of other factors. Many of the factors influencing food choice have their effects by changing an individual's attitudes towards the food. These attitudes may concern the sensory properties of the food, the health or nutritional value of the food or other characteristics of the food, such as its price or value for money. Attitudes towards foods are assumed to reflect the influence of many of these factors upon food choice (Shepherd 1989). In the social psychology of food we give particular attention to these psychological factors and their interaction with aspects of the food and the environment to help us to understand food choice and other food-related behaviours. Sensory differences between individuals in terms of sensitivity to and the acceptability of differing levels of the constituents in food will also influence food choices (Figure 1.1).

Differences in age, sex, social class, region of residence and degree of urbanization will also lead to differences in food consumption. These probably operate through some of the variables described above. Many of the variables will be interrelated and their effects difficult to distinguish. It should be noted that food choice is not a constant phenomenon, but will change with differing circumstances and experiences of the individual. In much of the remainder of the book the focus is upon the influences within the individual and how the food and the environment impact upon these influences to determine actual food choices and intake. These influences within the individual are social psychological variables, such as attitudes.

What should be clear from these examples is the fact that many of the influences upon food choices can be seen as operating through effects on individuals' attitudes. When these differing influences upon food choices are compared within an individual the major determinant of consumption is the flavour or taste of the food, with physiological factors like tolerance and satiety sometimes important, but beliefs about the healthiness of the food much less important and factors such as price and convenience having little or no effect on consumption (Shepherd 1989, 1999).

Overview of the content of this book

The remainder of this book is split into chapters examining specific topics within the domain of the social psychology of food. Rather than being exhaustive, the topics have been selected as areas within which the contribution of social psychological approaches has been particularly important, in our view. For each topic we have attempted to provide a general overview of a range of research within this area and then a more focused consideration of the contribution of social psychological approaches to furthering our understanding of the aspect of food being reviewed.

Taking the framework presented in Figure 1.1 as a starting point, Chapter 2 considers the question of why people eat the foods they do. Beginning with a look at the sensory and biological influences on food choice (and the way in which the two interact), we go on to argue that these processes are best understood in the context of the social world. The remainder of Chapter 2 examines the particular contribution of social psychology to our understanding of food choice, with a particular focus on the contribution of attitude theory to predicting food choice.

Chapter 3 considers health-related dietary change. While there are many reasons why people might want to change their diet, health is an important one. We begin by reviewing evidence on the relationship between diet and health, focusing in particular on attempts to reduce morbidity and mortality from cardiovascular diseases and cancer. We then review a number of social psychological models that have been used to predict dietary change, and go on to examine how such models can be used to change dietary intake. Finally, we consider the ways in which long-term dietary change might best be promoted.

In Chapter 4 we examine the important issues of weight control and disorders of eating. Body shape concerns and health outcomes are an important basis of efforts to control one's weight. We highlight the importance of social pressure as a key determinant of the desire for slim body shapes prevalent in most Western societies. The chapter examines obesity and its treatment as an extreme example of problems with weight control. We then review strategies employed to control weight. Social psychological research on the determinants of weight control behaviours is highlighted and given detailed consideration. Finally, the eating disorders of **anorexia** and **bulimia nervosa** are examined.

Chapter 5 focuses on the relationship between stress and eating. We define **stress** and show how it has been measured. The next section reviews work on the general effects of stress on eating. The major section of the chapter then reviews the individual difference approach to stress–eating relationships. This approach suggests that stress produces different effects (increased, decreased or no change) on eating in different groups. The major groups considered are the obese versus the non-obese, the restrained (i.e. dieter) versus the non-restrained and men versus women. In the next section we consider what research has taught us about the impact of stress on disordered eating. The final section considers a number of social psychological questions that this research poses. In particular, issues concerning the type and severity of the stress, which groups are affected, the types of food affected and the potential mechanisms are considered.

Chapter 6 deals with **social influences** on food intake. First, we examine the influence that the mere presence of others can exert on the amount we eat and the type of food we eat. Second, we investigate why and with whom these effects occur. Finally, we consider a number of the social psychological mechanisms that might explain these effects, notably the influence of **self-presentation** on the foods we eat.

Chapter 7 examines a number of interesting directions for future research on the social psychology of food.

Summary

The social psychology of food is concerned with the contribution of social psychology to our understanding of an important aspect of everyday life, namely our interaction with food. Social psychology is particularly concerned with how our thoughts, feelings and behaviours are influenced by others. Social psychological variables are only one of a number of factors relevant to our interaction with food (Figure 1.1). Nevertheless, these variables appear important because of their status as proximal determinants of behaviour that appear to mediate the impact of many other more basic influences. In addition, social psychological variables can often be manipulated, offering a useful way to intervene to change behaviour that has become dysfunctional or harmful to the individual. In the case of food choice we demonstrated the relative impact of different variables and the centrality of social psychological variables. Our choice of food is influenced by many differing factors. Attributes both of the food and of the eating context are likely to have effects on food selection. These differing influences can be split into those attributable to the food, those linked to the environment and those located within the individual. Those attributable to the food are associated with its chemical and physical composition, while those linked to the environment include the price, the culture and availability. These sorts of influences only make sense in relation to individual physiology, sensory perceptions and psychological factors. Together they form a complex amalgam of influences that determine our choice of food. Subsequent chapters of this book go on to explore the impact of the social psychological variables on food choice (Chapter 2), dietary change (Chapter 3), weight/shape control (Chapter 4), the impact of stress on eating (Chapter 5) and the role of food in self-presentation (Chapter 6). The final chapter considers directions for future work on the social psychology of food.

Suggested further reading

Axelson, M.L. and Brinberg, D. (1989) *A Social-psychological Perspective on Food-related Behavior*. New York: Springer-Verlag.

This is an excellent early review of work on social psychological perspectives on food choice. Models of the impact of attitudes on behaviour are given particularly detailed treatment.

Booth, D.A. (1994) *Psychology of Nutrition*. London: Taylor & Francis.

This book presents an individual and insightful review of research across a broad range of topics in the domain of nutrition, with a focus on the author's own contributions.

Capaldi, E.D. (ed.) (1996) *Why We Eat What We Eat: The Psychology of Eating*. Washington, DC: American Psychological Association.

This edited text brings together contributions from a number of key researchers in this area. Necessarily the focus is more upon physiological than social psychology.

Logue, A.W. (1991) *The Psychology of Eating and Drinking*, 2nd edn. New York: Freeman.

This is an easily accessible introduction to the broad field of eating and drinking.

Food choice

General overview

The study of food choice is principally concerned with one question: why do people eat the foods they do? On the surface, this may seem like a rather simple question, but the answer is often extremely complicated. After all, you don't necessarily have to be hungry, you don't *always* choose your most preferred option, and some of the influences might be unconscious. In our view, the study of food choice is *the* core topic in the social psychology of food, and issues raised in this chapter echo throughout the rest of the book. For example, some of the social psychological models of food choice we present in this chapter have been used as the basis for dietary change programmes (see also Chapter 3). Similarly, weight control (Chapter 4), perceived levels of stress (Chapter 5) and self-presentational **goals** (Chapter 6) all exert powerful influences upon the foods we choose to eat or choose to reject.

The central importance of the study of food choice has made it a correspondingly detailed field of study, with key scientific contributions being made by pharmacologists, physiologists, geneticists, economists and sociologists, as well as by psychologists. Using the overarching framework we presented in Chapter 1 (Figure 1.1), the following section examines sensory and biological influences on food choice and the way in which the two interact with the individual. We go on to argue that while sensory/biological influences are crucial to the development of a scientific account of food choice, these processes are best understood in the context of the social world. The bulk of the chapter therefore focuses on social psychological contributions to the understanding of food choice. The final section provides some directions for future research.

Sensory influences on food choices: experience versus innate preferences

The sensory perception of foods plays an important part in food choices. Most senses are important at some stage in food consumption (Shepherd and Farleigh 1989). For example, the visual appearance of a food is particularly important in stopping food consumption and may be used as a cue to ripeness or freshness (MacDougall 1987). Similarly, touch, sight and hearing are important in the perception of texture: particular types of texture are taken to be acceptable for different types of foods; for example, crunchy apples and creamy ice cream. However, taste and odour are the most important sensory factors in determining food choice. Odours can be perceived both before and after the food is placed in the mouth. Along with taste, odour forms part of the total perception of overall flavour. Taste is the perception of chemicals in the food mixed with saliva on the taste buds on the tongue. While there is little agreement as to the classification of odours, there are generally agreed to be four tastes: sweet (produced by substances such as sucrose), salty (produced by table salt and related substances), sour (from citric acid and similar compounds) and bitter (produced by substances such as caffeine).

We all know what our most and least favourite foods are and sometimes we can speculate on why. Research has been looking at what determines food preferences for some time. In terms of *sensory* differences in the food, the debate has for a long time revolved around the issue of whether preferences for certain sensory characteristics of foods are based upon our experiences with food or somehow determined by our genes (i.e. innate). Much of the research in this area has focused on our preference for tastes such as sweetness or saltiness. One way to study the relative importance of innate versus learned influences on food preferences is to examine the development of responses to foods. Presumably, the responses of newborns and infants should be little affected by the experiential factors that are likely to have a marked influence on adult preferences. This has led to much study of the newborn human infant to determine whether responses to sweetness and other basic tastes are innate.

The evidence from such research strongly points to an **innate preference** for sweet tasting substances. For instance, one study (Desor *et al.* 1973) found that infants aged between one and three days consumed more water the sweeter it was. Many researchers attribute this innate preference for sweetness to the fact that sweet sugars elicit the same reactions of pleasure in infants that they do in adults. A fascinating set of studies by Steiner (1977, 1979) supports this view. He gave newborn infants sugar solutions and photographed their reactions. The reaction to sweet tastes is characterized by a marked relaxation of many of the facial muscles, a slight smile and often licking and sucking of the tongue. This is in marked contrast to bitter and sour stimuli, which produce gaping or expulsive reactions in newborns. Steiner reports no marked differences in response between normal newborns of between three and seven days of age and those aged less than 20 hours (tested before their first feed). Hence, it is likely that preferences for sweet tastes over bitter or sour tastes are innate. Sweetness appears to be perceived as pleasant from birth, and higher levels are perceived as more pleasant, while bitter and sour tastes are perceived as unpleasant provided they are strong enough to taste. It may be that these preferences serve an evolutionary purpose. For instance, this innate responsiveness to sweetness may reflect an evolutionary pressure to ensure detection and recognition of food sources likely to be high in calories, while rejection of bitterness and sourness may indicate a pressure to avoid substances that are frequently inedible or even poisonous.

Analogous findings have been reported with respect to innate preferences for salt and milk and rejection of sour and bitter tastes (for a review see Birch 1999). However, this is not to say that genetic predisposition is the only influence on food preference; indeed, Birch (1999: 42) bemoans the 'widely accepted but erroneous view . . . that food preferences are unlearned, innate reflections of the body's need for nutrients'. In fact, most food preferences seem to be learned and are shaped by 'the context and consequences of eating . . . foods' (Birch 1999: 42). Congruent with this view, there is also evidence in support of the learned nature of sensory food preferences. For example, Beauchamp and Moran (1984) looked at three groups of children: those never fed sweetened water, those fed sweetened water for fewer than six months and those fed sweetened water for more than six months. At two years of age they were tested for their preferences for sweetened water, and only those groups who had been fed sweetened water showed a preference for sweetened over unsweetened water. Thus any innate preference for sweet tasting substances had become unlearnt and children only preferred what they were used to. Similarly, investigations into persons with a 'sweet tooth' have shown that preferences for high levels of sweetness occur across different food groups, suggesting that preference for sweet is learned rather than innate (Conner et al. 1988b; Conner and Booth 1988).

Another American study (Bertino et al. 1982) looked at the effects of adults changing their diet upon their subsequent food choices. A group of individuals made a large decrease in their overall dietary salt intake by cutting out many salty foods and no longer salting their food. Preferences for differing levels of salt in soup and crackers were subsequently assessed several months later and compared to those of a group who had not changed their diet. Those who had reduced their salt consumption were found to come gradually to prefer lower levels of salt in these two foods.

These studies suggest that any innate preferences for particular tastes may be subject to modification quite early in life. It seems likely that although we begin life with a preference for sweet foods and an aversion to bitter or sour tasting substances, our experience with differing foods and tastes leads us to prefer the normally experienced level of taste of the things we eat. That is to say, people come to prefer what they are used to and that this is likely to be a learned response.

The link between sensory characteristics of foods and the choice and consumption of foods has been an area greatly studied. Several authors suggest that sensory factors play a key role in determining food choice (Amerine *et al.* 1965). However, demonstrating a simple relationship between particular sensory characteristics and food choice is difficult, partly because sensory factors are but one of a range of influences upon individuals' food choices, all of which are operating simultaneously. Indeed, the studies reviewed above are all notable for the care they took to remove extraneous influences on behaviour. In less controlled environments, examining the relationship between sensory characteristics and consumption of a food is more difficult. One way in which this has been studied has been to argue that liking mediates the relationship between sensory factors and food choice. Thus, one can expose participants to various foods that differ in some sensory factor (such as sweetness) and then ask them to rate their liking for them. This particular approach has demonstrated that sensory differences in foods are linked to differences in liking. Unfortunately, there is not a perfect relationship between liking and food choice; for instance, while an individual might like chocolate, that does not mean to say she or he will select chocolate to eat at every meal.

More convincing is a method for examining the influences on food choice within an individual, which was developed by David Booth and colleagues (see Booth and Conner 1990; Conner and Booth 1992). This method involves presenting an individual with samples of a food varying in the characteristic of interest (e.g. level of salt) and observing corresponding variations in judgements about likelihood of choice. An individual psychophysical function relating the physical characteristic to choice in the individual is then developed (see Conner *et al.* 1986, 1988a,b; Conner and Booth 1988). The principal advantage of this approach is that it does not assume a perfect relationship between liking and food choice. However, given that these are exclusively laboratory-based studies, it may be difficult to extrapolate the findings to a general population, for whom sensation may be but one of a range of influences on food choice (e.g. Shepherd and Farleigh 1989).

Physiological influences on food choices

The function of the physiological system related to food intake is to regulate body weight, promote variety in diet and maintain an equilibrium. At a physiological level this can be seen as a feedback mechanism. Our eating behaviour determines our intake of nutrients that are essential to our functioning. One major objective of nutrition research is to study the ways in which the properties of foods influence their long-term pattern of consumption and so affect the health of the individual. The body must carefully balance the correct intake of calories and differing types of nutrients. The brain is 'informed' of the body's nutritional status and drives and directs our eating behaviour. Two main sets of physiological signals are responsible for the activation and termination of a meal. One set is thought to activate eating and is based principally upon the body's fat stores; when the fat stores, which contain the calories for physiological processes, fall below a certain level feelings of hunger are generated and eating takes place (Blundell and Rogers 1991). The powerful effect of feelings of hunger is clear to anyone trying to diet: reduced food consumption leads to strong feelings of a desire to eat, which often overwhelm and interfere with other activities (see Chapter 4). The second set of physiological signals are concerned with the termination of eating; these physiological signals give rise to feelings of satiety or fullness (Blundell and Rogers 1991). Together these two sets of factors help to ensure regular food intake designed to maintain a certain body weight.

The term hunger is used to refer to a drive or state of motivation, an impulsion to act. Hunger is also used to indicate a subjective experience or feeling that is associated with the desire to obtain and eat food. This subjective feeling of hunger includes physical sensations of the body or head, such as stomach emptiness or cramps, light-headedness, mild nausea, tightening of the throat and so on. Hunger feelings may be influenced by many different cues, such as the presence of food, the arrival of meal times and the stimulation of thoughts about food or eating. The actual feelings and events that stimulate the feelings of hunger can vary dramatically from one person to the next. What these feelings achieve is to stimulate thoughts about food and eating and so remind us that the body needs food. Eating food serves to remove these feelings at least temporarily. How does food achieve this effect?

The actual mechanisms involved in terminating eating can be divided into four categories – sensory-specific satiety, cognitive processes, post-ingestive processes and post-absorptive processes – in a mechanism sometimes called the **satiety cascade** (Blundell and Rogers 1991). Satiety is that state of inhibition over further eating which follows food consumption; it refers to an eating-induced decrease in eating motivation or the graded termination of eating. The satiating power of food refers to the capacity of food to suppress feelings of hunger and to remove the desire for further eating. The satiating power of food is therefore one important factor that limits the total amount of food consumed. These changes can involve both a temporary reduction in the palatability of some foods and the relief of bodily sensations labelled hunger. Like the individually preferred composition of familiar foods and drinks, all individual decisions to consume and to cease consuming on the basis of bodily sensations are learned. This learning sets up cognitive processes cued by sensory characteristics of the food or drink, physiological changes following ingestion of food and the environmental factors of time of day, servings, the behaviour of others etc. Of the metabolic changes, energy production in the liver is likely to have a fundamental controlling influence on satiety (Booth 1972). Thus the fact that certain foods possess greater satiating power than other foods can be learnt by individuals, and this becomes yet another factor influencing food choices. Moreover, these four factors influencing the termination of eating occur at different time points, meaning that each can exert subtle influence upon food choice.

The first process leading to satiety is a sensory effect. This is generated through the smell, taste, temperature and texture of food, and helps to bring eating to an end and inhibit eating of foods with similar sensory characteristics in the short term. These effects are embodied in the idea of *sensory-specific satiety*, which can be best explained by reference to how it has been studied. In one study (Rolls *et al.* 1981), participants rated the pleasantness of the taste of eight foods and then consumed as much of the foods as they liked. Two minutes after the end of this meal the subjects re-rated the taste of the eight foods. The perceived pleasantness of the food consumed in the meal decreased significantly more than that of the foods not eaten in the meal. Thus satiety appeared to be specific to the food that had been consumed. It was also found that this 'sensory-specific' (i.e. food stimulus-specific or cognitive) satiety caused less of the same food to be consumed in a subsequent meal, while having no effect on the consumption of very different foods. It has also been found that, in addition to reducing the pleasantness of the food consumed, there is also an interaction between foods, so that similar foods also show decreases in pleasantness. For instance, after the consumption of a sweet food, other sweet foods declined in pleasantness, while savoury foods were unaffected, whereas the consumption of savoury food decreased the pleasantness of other savoury foods, but not of the sweet foods (Rolls *et al.* 1984). Thus stimulus-specific satiety will limit the consumption of one type of food within a meal and may promote the consumption of a nutritionally varied diet, unless many powerful sensory differences are introduced into basically the same food type.

The second component of the satiety cascade concerns cognitive effects. These are the **beliefs** held about the properties of the foods and about their presumed effects upon the eater. So, for instance, certain foods are expected to be filling and to make you satiated. This may be learned from previous experience with the food item or may be a belief based upon the way in which a food product is advertised or talked about. Similarly, while best physiological evidence suggests that hunger and eating are not determined by deviations in energy resources from a 'set point', most people *believe* this is the case, implying that people are in danger of consistently overeating when they feel hungry (see Assanand *et al.* 1998). Whatever the source, it is clear that we carry round with us quite powerful beliefs about the appropriateness of particular portion sizes for differing foods. These beliefs may well lead us to expect to feel satiated after consuming particular portion sizes of particular foods in particular circumstances (e.g. eating larger portions of the same food in the evening than at lunch time).

A third set of influences upon satiety identified in the satiety cascade are post-ingestive processes. These include a number of possible actions, including stomach distension and rate of stomach emptying, the release of hormones from the duodenum and the stimulation of receptors along the intestine. All of these post-ingestive processes are thought to provide feedback about the impact of the food and so inhibit further eating. The fourth and final components of the satiety cascade are labelled post-absorptive effects. These include the effects of food once it has been absorbed into the blood stream, as well as the action of chemicals such as glucose and amino acids on receptors in the brain and body. It should be noted that the effects of each of these four stages will overlap and combine to produce an overall effect. It is also true that individuals can learn associations between particular sensory characteristics and their post-ingestive and post-absorptive effects, and control satiety in this way. Thus the number of calories in particular foods will affect the amount eaten via sensory cues and learning of the physiological effects of consumption.

Biopsychological and sociopsychological approaches to food choice

The previous sections briefly reviewed sensory and physiological influences on food choice. Clearly, any scientific analysis of food choice must be able to account for the underlying physiological mechanisms, such as innate preference, nutrient-specific appetites and learned food aversions. However, we would argue that research on a social level will provide the best explanation of food choice. This view is supported by a number of biological psychologists, who have suggested that the impact of physiology on food choice is probably mediated by social influences (e.g. Rogers and Blundell 1990; Birch 1999). Moreover, some of the cornerstones of biopsychological approaches to food choice are less widely supported than previously thought. For example, the evidence supporting specific regulatory mechanisms is weak (with the exception of salt and water); evidence for innate taste preference is equivocal; and learned food aversions account for only a minority of food choices. Indeed, Rogers and Blundell (1990: 35) conclude: 'Often, food choice will be guided by an individual's conscious appraisal of the likely after-effects of consuming a particular food' (see above). Therefore, although there is a clear role for underlying physiology in food choice: any effects are likely to be mediated by social influences, such as the decision-making processes studied by social psychologists. Further, Rogers and Blundell (1990: 38) argue that 'social factors may be *particularly* important in influencing the development of preferences for foods' (emphasis added), suggesting that social psychology may provide a particularly important account of human food choice. Support for this view is provided by evidence from the limited influence of pharmacotherapeutic dietary interventions (see Chapter 3) and studies which show that social psychological variables mediate the effects of physiology on behaviour (see below).

There is a growing body of evidence suggesting that physiological determinants of food choice are mediated by social psychological variables such as attitudes. For example, Bagiella *et al.* (1991) tested the influence of a number of drugs thought to inhibit dietary intake in obese patients. Of particular interest here, Bagiella *et al.* found that attitudes towards nutrition were influenced by 5-hydroxytryptophan, *d*-fenfluramine and fluoxetine, but not placebo, fenfluramine or fluvoxamine. More importantly, each of these drugs had specific effects on attitudes, providing powerful evidence in support of the idea that psychological variables mediate physiological influences on behaviour. Consistent with the work of Bagiella and colleagues, Teff and Engelman (1996: 567) presented data which 'suggest that the sensory attributes of food may play less of a role in modulating CPIR [cephalic phase insulin release] than an individual's psychological attitude towards food.' CPIR is a post-ingestive factor concerned with the release of insulin that occurs in response to food intake and has been researched extensively as a mechanism for moderating food intake. As such, Teff and Engelman (1996) hypothesized that the levels of insulin associated with CPIR would increase with palatable, but not with non-palatable, foods. Participants were 'sham fed' (i.e. tasted, chewed and then expectorated[1]), but no difference was found between palatable and non-palatable foods. However, there was a strong correlation between attitude to food and insulin release: those with more restrained attitudes towards food produced a greater CPIR. These studies show the importance of conscious appraisals as mediators of physiological mechanisms and the potential for such appraisals to determine food choice.

The relationship between physiological and psychological processes is also demonstrated by research on food aversions. Most of us have stories about how consumption of one particular food was followed by illness and now we cannot eat that food; indeed, the sight or smell of that particular food makes us feel nauseous. This effect has been demonstrated numerous times in both human and non-human animal studies and appears to be a simple learning process that is easy to acquire but one that is extremely powerful and difficult to overcome (Pelchat and Rozin 1982; Rozin 1990).

More generally, the work of Paul Rozin and colleagues (e.g. Rozin and Fallon 1987) has focused on the psychological appraisals that underpin the rejection of certain foods. Rozin and Fallon (1987) argue that there are three main motivations for rejecting foods: sensory-affective, anticipated consequences and ideation. Sensory-affective beliefs are concerned with the belief that a food item possesses negative sensory properties (e.g. smells or tastes bad); anticipated consequences are beliefs about the possible harmful outcomes of eating certain foods (e.g. vomiting, cancer, social ridicule); and ideation is knowledge about the origin or nature of foods. Each of these three motivations probably has its roots in the evolutionary need to avoid eating harmful and poisonous substances. Interestingly, both sensory-affective beliefs and beliefs about anticipated consequences are regarded as being common in most (human and non-human) animals, while ideation is likely to be uniquely human and largely fostered by culture (Rozin and Fallon 1987).

The importance of these three motivations is perhaps best demonstrated with reference to Rozin and Fallon's (1987) taxonomy of food rejection, which distinguishes between distasteful, dangerous, inappropriate and disgusting foods. First, *distaste* is regarded as a sensory-affective reaction to foods that are generally regarded as edible within a culture, but are not preferred by the individual. Second, *danger* is concerned with negative anticipated consequences and probably has its basis in the evolutionary need to avoid eating harmful and poisonous substances, but might also include individual allergic reactions to food. Third, *inappropriate* foods are those that are not regarded as food within a particular culture (e.g. stones, banana skins). Fourth, *disgust* stems from inferences about the nature or origin of an item, which are culturally determined; for example, faeces is regarded as universally disgusting among adults (Rozin and Fallon 1981). The implication is that food rejection (and thereby food choice) has both a biological and a social (cultural) basis: both human and non-human animals can reject foods on the basis of distaste and/or danger, but only humans can choose food on the basis of appropriateness or disgust.

Thus, while exposure to food items is clearly linked to food preferences, exposure is itself a function of cultural norms (Rozin 1990: Chapter 6). Individuals are only exposed to those foods that their culture supports. For instance, stones and banana skins are not considered to be food in most Western cultures and so exposure to stones and banana skins as food is minimal. The work of Paul Rozin and colleagues provide a framework for understanding the processes by which individuals reject certain classes of food, and boundary conditions for the kinds of foods that people are prepared to eat within a given culture. Beyond this, though, how do individuals choose which foods to eat?

Consistent with the work of Rozin and colleagues, beliefs and feelings about the effects of consuming particular foods are also important in determining consumption (Rozin and Fallon 1987). We believe that certain foods are more likely to make us overweight than others, or that some foods are more unhealthy than others. These beliefs have a role to play in determining our choice of foods. Most research on the effect of health beliefs on food consumption attempts to measure how strongly the individual thinks consuming that food item will lead to a particular outcome (e.g. 'It will make me fat') and also how much that outcome is valued (e.g. 'I don't want to get fat'). So, for instance, in looking at milk consumption we might look at the outcome 'increases my cholesterol' and also at how important cholesterol levels are for that individual. When measured in this way, health beliefs have been found to be an important determinant of certain food choices (Shepherd 1989). This influence is reflected in the way in which many foods are now being advertised as 'healthy' or 'good for you'. And, given the increasing concerns about the effects of our diet on our health, such health beliefs are likely to be increasingly important in determining the foods we choose.

The emotional basis of attitudes towards foods is also reflected in preferences or liking for particular foods. For example, consider Zajonc's (1968) **mere exposure** effect, whereby repeated exposure to (almost) any object results in greater liking for that object. Food preference is therefore likely to be at least partly based upon a mere exposure effect: we come to like what we are used to. Evidence to support this claim has been provided by the work of Leann Birch and colleagues, who have conducted research into **neophobia** (for a review see Birch 1999). Neophobia in food concerns the avoidance of new foods, something that represents a significant problem for many parents and can actually inhibit dietary variety in children. Birch and Marlin (1982) tested two-year-old children and found that repeated exposure to foods (i.e. tasting and eating) increased the children's preference for those foods. Thus, much of what we regard as food preference is probably simple exposure and, as much of it will happen during childhood, it will be based upon what foods were given to us at that time. It is also true that attitudes towards certain foods are learned by modelling what our parents do. For instance, studies have shown that children less than four years old will be more likely to taste an unfamiliar food if the adult present tastes the food first and particularly if the adult is the mother (Birch 1987). Moreover, even among young children social approval is one way in which the eating of new foods is encouraged: children's preferences for novel foods are increased by seeing their peers choose to eat them (Birch 1980).

However, we can then ask: what causes us to try particular foods in the first place? In fact, there is now a large body of research into parental influences on children's food preferences. For instance, repeatedly giving a child food while being very friendly increases the child's preference for the food (Birch *et al.* 1980). In contrast, rewarding a child for eating disliked foods (e.g. green vegetables) leads to further decreases in preference for these foods because the child learns that you must be rewarded to eat these foods and therefore they must be unpleasant (Birch *et al.* 1984). However, parental conceptions of what is 'healthy' are often at odds with government recommendations that emphasize the need for children to consume a varied diet. In fact, the evidence suggests that people in general tend to categorize foods as being 'good' or 'bad' and have a tendency to coerce children into consuming 'good' foods while restricting intake of 'bad' foods (e.g. Rozin *et al.* 1996; Birch 1999). These early social pressures are likely to exert long-lasting effects on beliefs concerning dietary intake.

Psychological influences on food choices

The evidence would therefore suggest that although physiological processes are fundamental to the understanding of food choice, they are likely to exert only an indirect impact on behaviour. Social psychological variables, such as attitudes (e.g. Teff and Engelman 1996) or an 'individual's conscious appraisal of the likely after-effects of consuming a particular food' (Rogers and Blundell 1990: 35), provide insight into the proximal determinants of food choice. This account does not deny the influence of physiology on food choice, but argues that its effects are mediated through social psychological variables, such as attitudes and beliefs. The implication is that study of such variables may uncover more proximal (and more modifiable: see Chapter 3) determinants of food choice. The remainder of the chapter concentrates on social psychological research into food choice and models of how social psychological variables influence choice.

In common with other branches of psychology, social psychological research into food choice has its roots in animal research on learning theory. Through systematic study of animal behaviour, both Herrnstein's matching law and optimal foraging theory have been developed as normative models of food choice. While these models have been successfully applied to some human food choice behaviours, it is the exclusively human models of behavioural decision-making (as applied to food choice) that have provided social psychologists with the greatest wealth of information concerning human food choice. The following section considers Herrnstein's matching law and optimal foraging theory before considering influential models of human behavioural decision-making.

Herrnstein's matching law

Herrnstein's (1961, 1970) work was principally based upon observations of pigeons. His **matching law** is based on the premise that animals (non-human and human) seek to maximize success in obtaining food. At the most basic level, it is designed to account for the fact that if a pigeon is rewarded every time it pecks a red button twice, or pecks a blue button once, it is more likely to peck the blue button. The differential rates of pecking to receive a reward are known as 'patterns of reinforcement': these patterns must be learned in order for the animal to receive reward. Once these patterns of reinforcement have been learned the animal matches its choices to those patterns of reinforcement. The goal of studies into the matching law has been to see whether the distribution of choices maps on to the distribution of reinforcement. Research in this area typically manipulates the pattern of reinforcement and examines any effects on the choices that are made.

Herrnstein's (1970) matching law can be illustrated by the following equation, which is based on the presence of two potential reinforcers. Herrnstein regarded the amount of reinforcement (i.e. the intrinsic value of the reinforcement) and the delay in receiving that reinforcement as central to food choice. In the equation below, the number of times a particular food is chosen (FC_1 and FC_2) is determined by the size of the rewards (S_1 and S_2) and the delay in receipt of those rewards (D_1 and D_2).

$$\frac{FC_1}{FC_2} = \frac{S_1}{S_2} \times \frac{D_2}{D_1}$$

Thus, imagine that a chicken may obtain corn from either the farmhouse (FC_2) or the chicken run (FC_1), and that 5 g of corn (S_1) is available every 4 hours (D_1) from the chicken run, but 10 g of corn (S_2) is available from the farmhouse every 7 hours (D_2). This would be expressed as:

$$\frac{FC_1}{FC_2} = \frac{5}{10} \times \frac{7}{4} = \frac{7}{8}$$

That is, the odds of the chicken choosing the farmhouse (FC_2) over the chicken run (FC_1) are 8 to 7. In terms of maximizing success in obtaining food, the chicken would therefore tend to choose the farmhouse as the 'safer' bet because, overall, the reinforcement is greater and the delay shorter.

This formula has been used to predict the food choices of a number of species, as well as to examine self-control in children (e.g. Davison and McCarthy 1988; Mischel *et al.* 1989). More recently, the theory has been expanded to take inter-species differences, human age group and reinforcer quality into account (e.g. Tobin and Logue 1994). However, while Herrnstein's matching law provides a useful model of food choice in some animals, it provides an incomplete account of food choice. Possible delay and size of reward are obvious influences on food choice, but what if the chicken judged that farmhouse corn was more palatable than corn near its run? By the same token, the costs and benefits associated with human food choices are rarely as clear-cut or malleable. Optimal foraging theory represents one attempt to extend Herrnstein's matching law and to address these limitations.

Optimal foraging theory

The basic premise of **optimal foraging theory** is that food choice is dependent upon gaining maximum input for minimum expenditure. Thus, while (human or non-human) animals seek to maximize their benefits, they seek simultaneously to minimize their costs. Clearly, costs and benefits in this sense are not usually monetary and might include distance travelled, inherent danger, nutritional value or even social standing. One of the strengths of the theory is that it can account for a wide variety of food choice behaviours: pandas are concerned only with obtaining bamboo and therefore only need to obtain an energy balance by finding the requisite amount of bamboo at the correct time. In contrast, humans must maintain their energy balance as well as considering (for example) their food preferences and vitamin and mineral intake (i.e. a 'balanced' diet).

In its most basic form, the theory takes into account: (a) the amount of effort involved in readying the prey for consumption (e.g. killing, stripping); and (b) the net energy gained (i.e. gross energy gained minus gross energy expended). The relative worth of obtaining one kind of food over another is determined by dividing net energy by effort: the chosen food is that which gives the best ratio. Optimal foraging theory is considered to provide a useful account of the behaviour of a number of different species (e.g. Pulliam 1974).

However, it is not regarded as ethical to test optimal foraging theory directly in individual humans, as any experiment would consist of directly manipulating the food intake and energy expenditure of humans. Despite this, anthropologists have used optimal foraging theory as a model to predict patterns of behaviour in groups of humans. For example, Zeleznik and Bennett (1991) studied the Bari hunters of Venezuela and found a strong association between predictions based on optimal foraging theory and the actual behaviour of the hunters. Similarly, archaeologists have applied optimal foraging theory to the study of prehistoric foraging. For example, Broughton (1994) examined prehistoric declines in the abundance of large mammals in Late Holocene California. Applying an updated version of optimal foraging theory, Broughton was able to identify human predatory activity as the most likely cause of this decline.

Both matching law and optimal foraging theory were developed through observation of and experimentation with non-human animal behaviour. As such, they provide useful models for the study of food gathering within non-human animals. Moreover, the models provide a framework within which to study human behaviour, although this work has predominantly been focused on pre-industrial societies (e.g. Zeleznik and Bennett 1991; Broughton 1994). Essentially, both models seek to specify the units of analysis for a cost–benefit analysis of acting to secure food: the matching law focuses upon maximizing the acquisition of food; optimal foraging balances effort expended with food gained. For humans in industrialized nations, expenditure of effort is likely to be just one in a range of potential constraints on food consumption. If one considers that the majority of people living in Western Europe have ready access to either public transport or a car, the effort expended between choosing a tin of baked beans over a tin of spaghetti hoops is likely to be negligible. Moreover, while preference for pulses as opposed to pasta is likely to exert some influence on the choice of one over the other, there are a range of other influences, including economic, cultural, social, health, availability and personal resources (both physical and psychological). In a sense, the matching law and foraging theory focus on the wrong kind of cost–benefit analysis: both models address only a narrow range of potential influences upon food choice and focus on calculations of *actual* cost and benefit. In contrast, social psychological models of food choice are more concerned with *perceived* costs and benefits. The remainder of this chapter focuses on social psychological models of behavioural decision-making that have been applied in the domain of food choice. While the fundamental notion of maximizing rewards and minimizing costs is retained from the animal models, these behavioural decision-making models allow for a greater range of influences on human food choice.

Expectancy-value theory

In contrast with Herrnstein's matching law and optimal foraging theory, **expectancy-value theory** (e.g. Edwards 1954; Peak 1955; Fishbein 1967a) is a model of *human* decision-making. That is, while expectancy-value (EV) theory has been influenced by research into animal behaviour, research has focused on explaining human behaviour. More importantly, EV theory was designed to explain decision-making in general, rather than food choice *per se*. This level of generality opens up this model to consider a range of potential influences on food choice, rather than simply the ratio of effort expended to food energy consumed.

Comparable with the matching law and optimal foraging theory, EV theory is based on the assumption that individuals are motivated to maximize the chances of desirable outcomes occurring and minimize the chances of undesirable outcomes occurring. Given a choice between two objects, individuals will choose the one that is associated with the most desirable outcome (i.e. the one that is *evaluated* most positively). This global **evaluation** (*attitude*) is derived from the perceived likelihood of the object possessing a number of key attributes (e.g. outcomes associated with purchasing a product), weighted by the evaluation of those outcomes. Note that sensory-affect beliefs and anticipated consequences from Rozin and Fallon's (1987) model of food rejection could be interpreted as being negative outcomes associated with consuming particular foods.

Perhaps the most influential advocate of EV theory in social psychology has been Martin Fishbein. In his summative model of attitudes, Fishbein (1967a, b) argued that individuals may possess a large number of beliefs about a particular object, although only a subset of these are likely to be salient at any one time (see also Ajzen 1996; Ajzen and Fishbein 2000). Thus, attitudes towards objects (e.g. behaviours, products) are proposed to be determined by *salient* underlying beliefs computed by multiplying (weighting) the perceived likelihood of salient outcomes occurring with the value attached to those particular outcomes. The formal equation is:

$$Attitude = \sum_{i=1}^{n} b_i e_i$$

where b refers to the outcome belief and e refers to the evaluation of that belief, which when multiplied together are referred to as **behavioural beliefs**, i represents a particular attribute and n represents the number of attributes salient at any one time. The salient beliefs are then summed to produce an overall evaluation, or attitude. By way of an example, in choosing between cheese A and cheese B, a consumer might judge the likelihood of the cheeses having a strong flavour and a long shelf-life, and being a recognized brand. These judgements would then be weighted by the evaluation of each of these attributes (e.g. is strong flavour good or bad; is the shelf-life good or bad; is the brand good or bad?) and summed to provide an overall evaluation. If the consumer values strongly flavoured cheese with a short shelf-life and a recognized brand name *and* perceives that cheese A is more likely to possess these qualities than cheese B, she or he is more likely to choose cheese A. By the same token, if the **attitude object** is a behaviour (e.g. eating a low-fat diet), the individual might rate the likelihood that (for example) eating a low-fat diet will reduce the risk of heart disease, will be tasty and will reduce weight before positively or negatively evaluating each outcome. Again, the sum of these beliefs will provide an overall attitude towards eating a low-fat diet that will be compared with not eating a low-fat diet. The course of action that is evaluated the most positively is the one that is most likely to be pursued. At this point, it should be noted that this approach to attitude formation is regarded as a representation, rather than a realistic description of the processes involved, as Ajzen and Fishbein (2000: 7–8) state: 'In actuality, although the investigator does perform these computation, people are *not* assumed to do so. We merely propose that attitude formation may be *modeled* in this fashion.'

As we have already pointed out, there are a number of possible outcomes associated with particular foods (e.g. putting on weight, whether it will satisfy hunger, feeling ill), but it is the beliefs that are *salient* at the time that are held to be important (Fishbein and Ajzen 1975). Beyond this, only a small percentage of human beliefs and attitudes towards foods result directly from our interaction with foods: many beliefs are derived from socially transmitted information. These include beliefs about which foods are healthy and unhealthy, which foods are generally acceptable and which are not. Thus, while some food choices are clearly based upon experience with food (e.g. taste aversions), others are based upon the cultural meaning of food (e.g. the concern in Western culture with not eating too much is clearly linked to the current culturally ideal slim body shape for both men and women).

Although the EV model is one of general behavioural decision-making, it provides some insight into the kinds of psychological processes that influence human food choice decisions. A number of studies have investigated this. For example, Towler and Shepherd (1992) interviewed 34 people about the outcomes they associated with eating four food groups that have been associated with excessive fat intake: meat, meat products, dairy products and fried foods. From these interviews, salient outcomes about each of the food groups were elicited, three of which were identical across the food groups ('. . . is healthy', '. . . is high in fat', '. . . tastes good'). Other beliefs included 'expense' (meat and meat products), 'protein' (meat and dairy products) and 'convenience' (meat products and fried foods). Towler and Shepherd (1992) tested the ability of these beliefs to predict attitudes towards these food groups in a further sample of 240 individuals. Findings indicated that 'taste' and 'health' were important determinants of attitudes towards each food group, while 'fat' was predictive of only dairy products and fried foods. In addition, 'expense' and 'vitamins' were predictive of attitudes towards meat; and 'vitamins' was predictive of attitudes towards dairy products. Towler and Shepherd's (1992) study provides evidence to support the utility of the EV approach to understanding attitudes: different behavioural beliefs underpin attitudes to specific food groups.

Similar research has utilized the EV model to examine attitudes to whole diets. For example, eating a low-fat diet is a key UK government health target: given the serious health risks from excessive fat intake, it is recommended that individuals consume no more than 35 per cent of their food energy from fat in the diet (Department of Health 1992: Chapter 3). EV theory predicts that an individual's overall attitude to eating a low-fat diet will be determined by the salient outcomes associated with that behaviour. In a study conducted by Armitage and Conner (1999a) eight salient outcomes were identified through pilot interviews, of which four were predictive of attitudes towards eating a low-fat diet ('. . . makes me feel good about myself', '. . . reduces my enjoyment of food', '. . . helps to maintain a lower weight', '. . . eating fat makes me feel guilty'). Interestingly, behavioural beliefs that specified health outcomes (e.g. '. . . reduces my risk of coronary heart disease') were unrelated to attitudes. The implication is that appeals designed to change dietary intake via health appeals might be relatively ineffective compared with appeals to weight loss and the taste of low-fat alternatives.

While researchers typically take great pains to ensure that the behavioural beliefs they measure are salient within the target population, research by van der Pligt and de Vries (1998) suggests that the importance placed on beliefs is significant. Reasoning that more important beliefs are likely to be more salient, they asked individuals to nominate the three beliefs that they regarded as most important. The results are striking: the three most important beliefs were strongly correlated ($r = 0.63$) with overall attitude, in contrast with the correlation between the 12 less important beliefs and attitude ($r = 0.15$). Although van der Pligt and de Vries's study examined attitudes towards smoking, the inclusion of measures of belief importance might well enhance the predictive validity of the EV model (for a review of alternative approaches, see van der Pligt et al. 2000).

The research by Towler and Shepherd (1992) and Armitage and Conner (1999a) demonstrates the utility of the EV model for predicting food choice attitudes. This perspective extends those of the matching law and optimal foraging theory by capturing a range of potential influences on food choices. However, while it is clearly important to study the decision-making processes underpinning attitudes towards food, the real power of this approach lies in the ability of attitudes to predict actual food choice. After all, as noted by Ajzen and Fishbein (2000), the EV model presents an idealized form of decision-making that might not be conducted in everyday situations. The following section focuses on research that has investigated the proposed relationship between attitudes and behaviour.

The attitude–behaviour relationship

The social psychological study of attitudes has been one of the core areas of the discipline for decades, described by Allport (1935: 798) as 'probably the most distinctive and indispensable concept in contemporary . . . social psychology'. This concept has spawned a considerable amount of work in social psychology and has been defined in various ways (for reviews see Eagly and Chaiken 1993; Ajzen 2001). For example, Eagly and Chaiken (1993: 1) define an attitude as 'a psychological tendency that is expressed by evaluating a particular entity with some degree of favor or disfavor', and this evaluative response may be 'overt or covert, cognitive, affective, or behavioral'. As we have already seen, overt attitudes towards food have been shown to mediate the effects of biology on behaviour.

Commensurate with the amount of research attention directed at the attitude–behaviour relationship in general, many studies have examined this in conjunction with food choice. In fact, Conner (2000) identified a total of 143 tests of this relationship. Using meta-analysis, Conner (2000) found that correlations between food choice attitudes and behaviour were in the moderate ($0.21 < r < 0.40$) to large ($0.41 < r < 0.60$) range. This is directly comparable to the size of relationship ($0.30 < r < 0.49$) reported for the attitude–behaviour relationship in reviews of all behaviours (e.g. Kim and Hunter 1993; Kraus 1995). Hence this provides support for the study of attitudes as a strong correlate of food-related behaviours. However, these data hide the fact that the average frequency-weighted correlation between attitudes and behaviour was 0.35. While this figure equates with explaining more than 12 per cent of the variance in behaviour, clearly the correspondence between attitudes and behaviour is less than perfect. The two dominant approaches to explaining this lack of correspondence are outlined in the following section.

Thus far, we have assumed that attitudes are an important determinant of behaviour; intuitively, one might expect that individuals who have more positive attitudes towards certain types of food are more likely to consume those foods. A serious threat to this assumption came from Wicker's (1969) review of the attitude–behaviour link and his conclusion that, at best, only a weak correlation connected expressed attitudes and behaviour. There were two main responses to the perceived threat. The first was a consideration of various moderating factors; in other words, an examination of variables that affect the *relationship* between attitudes and behaviour, such as imprecise measurement or the strength of attitude. The second was the exploration of mediating variables, or the idea that the influence of attitudes on behaviour is actually indirect, filtered through some other variable (for further discussion of this moderating–mediating distinction see Baron and Kenny 1986).

Measurement issues and the attitude–behaviour relationship

Fishbein and Ajzen's (1975) **principle of correspondence** stems from the finding that attitudes are most predictive of behaviour when the two measures are congruent with respect to action (e.g. eating), target (e.g. an apple), time (e.g. this afternoon) and context (e.g. during a meeting). Thus, the principle of correspondence states that in order to maximize the relationship between attitude and behaviour, one must measure both components with similar levels of specificity. For the example provided above, an individual's attitude might be measured using an item such as:

My eating an apple during this afternoon's meeting would be

Negative   −3   −2   −1   0   +1   +2   +3   Positive

Her or his behaviour should be measured at a similar level of specificity (e.g. did I eat an apple during my meeting this afternoon?). Clearly, this level of specificity is likely to maximize the relationship between attitudes and behaviour (for a review see Ajzen and Fishbein 1977), but is unlikely to provide useful information about the behaviour of any other people. It is also questionable how interesting apple-eating-in-meetings-behaviour actually is! However, the principle of correspondence allows for the prediction of more general behaviours by emphasizing the fact that it is the *correspondence* between measures that is important, rather than the level of specificity. In short, general attitudes should be more predictive of a general measure of behaviour than a specific attitude. For example, a healthy eating attitude could be measured by responses to the following item:

My eating a healthy diet in the next 12 months would be

Negative   −3   −2   −1   0   +1   +2   +3   Positive

A year-long assessment of dietary intake in the same individual would provide a measure of behaviour at a suitable level of correspondence, and one might expect a reasonable attitude–behaviour correlation across individuals. In contrast, this measure of attitude is unlikely to be predictive of a one-off measure of apple eating in meetings.

Support for the principle of correspondence has been considerable, and has been widely applied both within and outside social psychology (e.g. Ajzen and Fishbein 1977). Conner's (2000) meta-analysis confirmed this, reporting that measures showing good levels of correspondence in relation to action and target produced stronger attitude–behaviour correlations ($r = 0.40$ versus 0.33). Hence, researchers examining attitude as a predictor of food behaviours would be well advised to ensure good correspondence in their different measures.

Despite this, attitudes are generally found to be better predictors of specific behaviours than more general classes of behaviours or goals. This effect was partially supported in Conner's (2000) review. For the attitude–behaviour relationship, the correlation was stronger for specific foods ($r = 0.44$) and dietary constituents ($r = 0.38$) than for general aspects of the diet ($r = 0.28$), irrespective of the principle of correspondence. Hence, more specific behaviours appear to be better correlated with attitudes and one might recommend a focus on more specific behaviours. It has been suggested that this effect is attributable to the fact that attitudes are more likely to be causal determinants of a specific action. In contrast, more general classes of behaviours (or goals) might be achieved in a number of different ways, meaning that a range of other factors are likely to be important in addition to the general attitude (or goal attitude). For example, healthy eating may be achieved by reducing fat intake, increasing fruit and vegetable consumption, decreasing salt intake and/or reducing snacking, some of which may be more acceptable to an individual than others. In such a case, the attitudes towards different means of achieving the goal may be the better predictor (see Conner and Norman 1996; see also Chapter 4). We return to this issue later.

Indirect effects of attitudes on behaviour

A second strand of Fishbein and Ajzen's (1975) work has actually suggested an *indirect* link between attitudes and behaviour, proposing **behavioural intention** as a mediating variable. Behavioural intention was defined as the motivation required to perform a particular behaviour: the more one intended to perform a behaviour, the more likely would be its performance. Explicit within these conceptualizations is the causal link between salient (behavioural) beliefs, attitudes, intention and behaviour, respectively. Support for this view is reported by the meta-analysis of Conner (2000), who found that the overall frequency-weighted correlation between attitudes and behaviour ($r = 0.35$) was significantly weaker than either the attitude–intention ($r = 0.46$) or the intention–behaviour relationship ($r = 0.43$). The implication is that the indirect impact of attitudes on behaviour via intentions is greater (0.20) than the direct effect (0.15). This is partial support for behavioural intentions as mediators of the attitude–behaviour relationship. More direct evidence is provided by studies into the theories of reasoned action and planned behaviour, which include measures of attitude and behavioural intention within a broader theoretical framework.

The theory of reasoned action

The behavioural beliefs, attitude, intention and behaviour model forms the basis of Fishbein and Ajzen's (1975) **theory of reasoned action** (see also Ajzen and Fishbein 1980). In addition, the theory of reasoned action (TRA) proposes a second determinant of intention: **subjective norms**. Subjective norms are defined as perceptions of general social pressure to perform or not to perform a given behaviour. Underlying subjective norms are **normative beliefs**: the perceived social pressure from salient referents weighted by an individual's **motivation to comply** with those referents. For example, one might perceive social pressure from one's parents to eat cabbage, but this

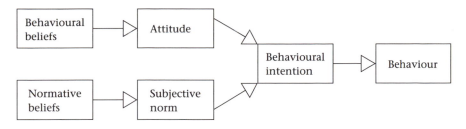

Figure 2.1   The theory of reasoned action

social pressure will only be influential to the extent that one is motivated to comply with one's parents. Congruent with behavioural beliefs, salient normative beliefs are held to determine subjective norms. A schematic representation of the TRA is presented in Figure 2.1.

Several quantitative and narrative reviews have provided support for use of the TRA in the prediction of a number of behaviours (e.g. Sheppard *et al.* 1988; van den Putte 1991). More specifically, the model has been used to predict both specific and more general food choices. For example, Saunders and Rahilly (1990) used the TRA to predict the reduction of fat and sugar consumption in students who were either majoring in health studies or not majoring in health studies. Taking the sample as a whole, both attitude and subjective norm were predictive of intentions, accounting for 41 per cent of the variance. Interestingly, when the sample was divided into health majors and non-health majors, attitudes were the dominant predictors of the intentions of health majors, whereas subjective norms were the dominant predictors of non-health majors. The implication is that the health majors were more knowledgeable about the outcomes associated with reducing fat and sugar intake, making their decision to eat healthily less open to the influence of social pressure.

In another study, Anderson and Shepherd (1989) examined the ability of the TRA to predict 'healthier eating' in a sample of 95 women attending ante- and post-natal clinics. Again, the predictive validity of the model was supported, with attitude and subjective norm together accounting for 28 per cent of the variance in intentions. However, in this case, only attitude was a significant predictor: subjective norm did not exert a significant effect on the decisions of these women. Thus a number of applications of the TRA to food choice have provided support for the model. However, despite all the supporting evidence, Ajzen (1988: 127) himself concedes, 'The theory of reasoned action was developed explicitly to deal with purely volitional behaviors'; in other words, simple behaviours, where successful performance of the behaviour requires only the formation of an intention. The implication was that behaviours were solely dependent on personal agency (i.e. the formation of an intention), and that control over behaviour (e.g. personal resources or environmental determinants of behaviour) was relatively unimportant.

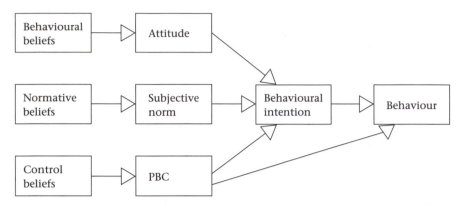

Figure 2.2 The theory of planned behaviour

The theory of planned behaviour

Ajzen (1988: 132) proposed 'a conceptual framework that addresses the problem of incomplete volitional control', which would address the limitations of the TRA: the **theory of planned behaviour** (Ajzen 1988, 1991). The theory of planned behaviour (TPB; see Figure 2.2) extended the TRA by including a measure of **perceived behavioural control** as a determinant of both intentions and behaviour. The inclusion of perceived behavioural control (PBC) as a predictor of behaviour is based on the rationale that holding intention constant, greater perceived control will increase the likelihood that enactment of the behaviour will be successful. Further, to the extent that perceived control reflects actual control, perceived behavioural control will directly influence behaviour. Perceived behavioural control therefore acts as both a proxy measure of actual control and a measure of confidence in one's ability.[2] Within the TPB, perceived behavioural control (PBC) is posited as a third determinant of intention: the easier a behaviour is, the more likely it is that one will intend to perform it. Congruent with the other belief components, salient **control beliefs** determine these global perceptions of control. Control beliefs are the perceived frequency of occurrence of facilitating or inhibiting factors multiplied by the perceived power of those factors to inhibit/facilitate the behaviour in question.

Applications of the TPB to food choice

A series of narrative and quantitative reviews (e.g. Ajzen 1991; van den Putte 1991; Conner and Sparks 1996; Godin and Kok 1996; Armitage and Conner 2001b) have shown the efficacy of the TPB in predicting behaviour in general. Sparks (1994) reviews applications of the TPB to food choice, which demonstrate that the PBC component makes a significant contribution to the predictive power of the TRA, providing support for the TPB.

More specifically, there have been several applications of the TPB to the prediction of food choice intentions, from the use of gene technology in food production (e.g. Sparks *et al.* 1995) to fat intake (e.g. Nguyen *et al.* 1996). For example, Cox *et al.* (1998) found that the TPB accounted for between 33 and 47 per cent of the variance in intentions to increase fruit and vegetable consumption, with attitude being the dominant predictor, followed by subjective norm and perceived behavioural control. Comparably, Nguyen *et al.* (1996) found that attitude, subjective norm and perceived behavioural control independently contributed to the prediction of the intention to eat fatty foods. The final model accounted for 51 per cent of the variance in intention.

Notably, Nguyen *et al.*'s (1996) study demonstrated that sociodemographic influences (e.g. age, gender) were mediated by the TPB. Thus, gender and age differences in fat intake were completely explained by TPB variables. Accumulated research evidence demonstrates that there are sociodemographic variations in dietary intake (e.g. Blaxter 1990). However, given that such variables are not generally amenable to change, researchers have attempted to identify those variables that explain the relationship between sociodemography and behaviour (e.g. TPB). Thus, Nguyen *et al.*'s (1996) finding is important because targeting such variables might facilitate dietary change (see also Chapter 3) and because it provides evidence to suggest that the TPB can account for a variety of external influences on food choice (cf. Chapter 1).

However, the studies reviewed thus far have focused attention on predicting behavioural intentions, rather than on actual food choice. Although this approach provides some insight into the influences on individuals' food choices, it would be more useful to know whether these influences carried forward to predicting actual behaviour. More powerful still would be a model that was predictive of behaviour over a period of some time. Our own work has attempted to conduct prospective studies that measure actual behaviour. For example, comparable with the work reviewed above, Povey *et al.* (2000) found that the TPB explained 57 per cent of the variance in intentions to eat five portions of fruit and vegetables. Importantly, Povey *et al.* (2000) assessed actual behaviour one month later, finding that the TPB accounted for 32 per cent of the variance in actual fruit and vegetable consumption.

Similarly, Armitage and Conner (1999a) conducted a study that asked participants about their attitudes and intentions towards eating a low-fat diet. These participants were contacted again after a month and asked whether or not they had eaten a low-fat diet in the intervening period. Analyses of these responses revealed that the TPB accounted for 39 per cent of the variance in behaviour. However, unlike fruit and vegetable consumption, where it is possible to count portions with at least some level of accuracy, it is harder for people to assess how much fat they have actually eaten in the past month. So, in addition to asking people to infer how much fat they had consumed in the previous month, we asked participants to complete a more objective measure of behaviour that has been validated by nutritionists (a food frequency questionnaire: see Cade and Margetts 1988; Margetts *et al.* 1989). Interestingly, this measure was only modestly correlated ($r = 0.37$) with the self-perception measure, providing support for the idea that people find it hard to judge accurately the fat content of their own diets. Consistent with this, the TPB was only able to account for 18 per cent of the variance in behaviour using this more objective measure of behaviour. The findings of Povey *et al.* (2000) and Armitage and Conner (1999a) raise a number of key applied and theoretical issues about this approach to understanding food choice, which we consider in the following sections.

Measuring behaviour

Armitage and Conner's (1999a) study found that the TPB accounted for considerably more of the variance in a subjective measure of behaviour than in the more objective measure, a finding that has been replicated many times and in a number of domains (see Armitage and Conner 2001b). Some authors have argued that individuals are responding in a socially desirable manner when asked to infer their own healthy eating behaviour. In other words, it has been argued that individuals seek to maintain a positive image in the eyes of others and seriously overestimate the extent to which they are healthy eaters (see Chapter 6 for further discussion of this issue). However, research suggests that individuals are actually unlikely to respond to dietary questionnaires in a socially desirable manner (see Armitage and Conner 1999b). On a conceptual level, the mismatch between subjective and objective measures of dietary behaviour might be attributable to breaches in the principle of correspondence (Fishbein and Ajzen 1975). The objective measure employed by Armitage and Conner (1999a) involves reporting about consumption of 63 individual items of food, whereas the subjective measure ('Did you eat a low-fat diet in the last month?') maps directly on to the measure of intention ('Do you intend to eat a low-fat diet in the next month?'). Clearly this presents something of a conundrum: how to achieve correspondence between a measure of intention and the more objective measure of behaviour. In fact, Sutton (1998) has proposed an elegant solution to this problem: that of showing participants the behaviour measure they will complete in the future before they report their intentions. Other commentators (e.g. Bagozzi 1992) have argued that it is unfair to relate people's intentions to their behaviour. After all, performance of a behaviour can be either successful or unsuccessful without the determining factors (e.g. attitudes, intentions) being any different. Bagozzi's (1992) theory of trying describes the influences upon the decision to try and actual trying to achieve a particular goal in order to circumvent these potential problems (see Chapter 4).

Consistent with Conner's (2000) review of the attitude–behaviour relationships within food choice research, it is clear that the TPB accounts for considerably more of the variance in specific dietary behaviours than more global dietary behaviours. Povey *et al.* (2000) showed that the TPB accounted for 32 per cent of the variance in fruit and vegetable consumption, compared with 18 per cent of the variance explained in Armitage and Conner's (1999a) low-fat diet study. As we argued above, this effect is attributable to the fact that specific actions are easier to predict because the number of ways of achieving them is, by definition, limited (for a review see Baranowski *et al.* 1999). In contrast, more general classes of behaviours (or goals), such as eating a low-fat diet, might be achieved in a number of different ways and it is likely that a range of factors will be important in addition to the general attitude (or goal attitude). By the same token, eating a low-fat diet is more complex than eating five portions of fruit and vegetables per day because there are more component behaviours (identifying high-fat foods, locating low-fat alternatives, purchasing appropriate foods etc.). The implication is that more complex models are required for more complicated behaviours and that for a goal such as eating a low-fat diet, one needs to assess a range of attitudes, rather than simply a global attitude to eating a low-fat diet.

Additional variables within the TPB

Notwithstanding the differences in the behaviours studied by Povey *et al.* (2000) and Armitage and Conner (1999a), it is clear that the TPB was less than perfect at predicting food choice. One clear goal for researchers has been to increase the proportion of variance explained in intentions and behaviour. A number of approaches have been adopted, most notably the inclusion of variables in addition to attitude, subjective norm and PBC. The inclusion of these additional variables is regarded as an effective way of accounting for more variance in intentions and behaviour.

Unusually in the field of social psychology, Ajzen (1991: 199) regards his TPB as being 'open to the inclusion of additional predictors if it can be shown that they capture a significant proportion of the variance in intention or behavior after the theory's current variables have been taken into account.' As such, recent research has focused on using the TPB as a framework for understanding the influence of a range of other social cognitive variables on intention and behaviour (e.g. Conner and Armitage 1998). Two variables in particular have attracted the attention of social psychologists: research into **self-identity** and **perceived need** are reviewed below.

Sparks (2000: 35) regards *self-identity* as being 'synonymous with self-perception or self-concept' and as referring 'to the relatively enduring characteristics that people ascribe to themselves'. Self-identity is held to exert motivational significance insofar as individuals seek to perform behaviours that maintain their sense of self. In food choice, one might be more likely to eat healthily if one sees oneself as 'health conscious' and to eat environmentally friendly foods if one is a 'green consumer'. A number of empirical investigations have supported the independent predictive power of self-identity. For example, Sparks and Shepherd (1992) found that self-identification as a 'green consumer' significantly contributed to the prediction of intentions to consume organically grown vegetables, over and above the effects of TPB variables. Related work has demonstrated effects in relation to eating a low-fat diet (Sparks and Guthrie 1998; Armitage and Conner 1999a) and eating a healthy diet (Armitage and Conner 1999b). Thus, the way in which one sees oneself exerts significant influence on the motivation to choose certain foods.

There are two explanations of the self-identity–intention relationship. First, Charng *et al.* (1988) argue that while models such as the TRA and TPB are predictive of people's behaviour, over time people are more motivated by their need to retain their sense of self than by their attitudes or by perceived social pressure. Thus, Charng *et al.* (1988) argue that repeated performance of a behaviour develops one's self-concept. Applying this to the Sparks and Shepherd (1992) study on green consumerism, the implication is that to the extent that the behaviour is repeated over time, one's intention to purchase organic foods will be driven solely by self-identity. The second explanation for the self-identity–intention relationship argues that individuals are motivated to communicate their values and identity to others (Katz 1960; Shavitt 1990). To extend this view to the Sparks and Shepherd (1992) paper, this implies that choosing organic food is a communicative act, designed to express one's credentials as a 'green consumer'. To date, it is unclear which provides the better account of the self-identity–intention relationship, but we return to the issue of food choice as communicative act in Chapter 6.

Paisley and Sparks (1998) have demonstrated that *perceived need* is an important predictor of intentions to eat healthily. These authors argue that while the TPB includes measures of individuals' overall evaluations, there is no assessment of whether individuals see themselves as *needing* to (for example) eat a low-fat diet. Paisley and Sparks (1998) have shown that perceived need adds significantly to the prediction of behavioural intentions, over and above the effects of TPB variables. More recently, Povey *et al.* (2000) reported that perceived need added 11 and 6 per cent to variance explained in intentions with respect to eating five portions of fruit and vegetables per day and eating a low-fat diet, respectively. However, given that perceived need is so closely related to behavioural intention ($r = 0.67, 0.73$: Povey *et al.* 2000), it is unclear whether the construct truly adds anything distinct to the TPB. Given that behavioural intention is regarded as a summary of the motivation required to engage in a particular behaviour, it is possible that perceived need might more usefully be incorporated in measures of intention. One way to address this issue would be to manipulate perceived need experimentally and so to attempt to dissociate it from effects on behavioural intention.

More generally, despite the contributions made by these two variables, the true value of their contribution is open to question. First, it is notable that each of these variables exerts its influence on actual food choice *indirectly*, via behavioural intentions. As discussed above, this approach can provide only a partial account of actual food choice: the challenge is to identify variables that exert direct influence on behaviour. Second, Conner and Armitage's (1998) meta-analysis indicates that, on average, self-identity explains only 1 per cent unique variance in intention. While meta-analytic data on perceived need are not currently available, it is clear that the variable contributes less to the prediction of intention than the components of the TPB. Third, the majority of studies that have tested the role of additional variables within the TPB have only investigated additive effects. That is, researchers typically statistically control for the effects of TPB variables before seeing whether the additional variable of choice explains significant additional variance. Very few studies have investigated interactive or moderator (see Baron and Kenny 1986) effects of additional variables, which might equally add to our understanding of food choice. For example, it is possible that self-identity might moderate the attitude–intention relationship such that the attitudes of high identifiers are more predictive of intentions than are those of individuals who do not identify themselves as (for example) green consumers. The potential contribution of this approach was demonstrated in a study of voting behaviour: Granberg and Holmberg (1990) demonstrated that the intentions of high identifiers were more predictive of behaviour than were the intentions of low identifiers.

Some food choice studies *have* tested moderator effects, although the focus has been upon investigating the *properties* of TPB variables rather than on variables that might add to the prediction of intention/behaviour. One property that has recently been investigated is that of temporal stability, or the idea that (for example) the attitudes of some individuals may be more stable over time and hence more predictive of intention and behaviour. In fact, this is one of the early assumptions of models like the TPB (e.g. Fishbein and Ajzen 1975) and, given that many studies assess TPB variables and behaviour several months apart, controlling for the (in)stability of components means that extraneous influences such as mass media campaigns, spontaneous changes in attitudes or exposure to uncontrolled health promotion materials can be accounted for. For example, Conner *et al.* (2000) found that more stable intentions were more predictive of eating a low-fat diet three months later. More recently, Conner *et al.* (2002) extended these findings by testing the predictive validity of the TPB across a six-year time period. Consistent with Conner *et al.* (2000), Conner *et al.* (2002) found that stable intentions were more predictive of an objective measure of healthy eating taken six years later than were unstable intentions. Stability is therefore one property that enhances the predictive power of behavioural intentions. Moreover, similar stability effects have been reported with respect to the influence of perceived behavioural control on behaviour (see Conner *et al.* 2000).

A second property that has been investigated is the extent to which individuals plan their future behaviour. Thus, in parallel with work on intention stability, a number of authors have focused on the 'gap' between cognition and action (e.g. Kuhl 1985; Gollwitzer 1993; Sheeran 2002). More specifically,

Gollwitzer (1993) has argued that practical (volitional) strategies such as **implementation intentions** are important in ensuring that cognitions such as intentions are translated into action. Implementation intentions are plans that ensure decisions are acted upon by specifying the conditions under which a target behaviour will be performed. Thus, asking individuals to form an implementation intention (e.g. 'I intend to eat fresh fruit when offered dessert') should increase the likelihood of them actually doing so. This prediction is supported by accumulated empirical evidence that demonstrates that the formation of implementation intentions facilitates the translation of cognition into action (for a review see Sheeran 2002). Verplanken and Faes (1999) used implementation intentions to encourage consumption of a healthy diet. They randomized participants to either an implementation intention condition or a control condition. The implementation intention intervention asked participants to choose a day on which they would eat healthily and then to plan exactly what they would eat and drink on that day. Individuals in the implementation intention condition reported eating significantly more healthily in the next week. Thus, Verplanken and Faes's (1999) study suggests that implementation intentions are a useful tool for promoting healthy eating. Crucially, the effects of implementation intentions occurred irrespective of whether participants habitually ate poor diets. Implementation intentions may therefore represent a useful tool for dietary change (see Chapter 3).

The third property of TPB variables that has been investigated is **attitude strength**, and stronger attitudes have been shown to be more predictive of intentions (e.g. Sparks *et al.* 1992). More recently, a number of social psychologists have considered the possibility that attitudes might be multi-dimensional. As we have already noted in our discussion of the EV model, attitudes towards objects are generally held to be summaries of decision-making processes. The implication is that individuals 'decide' whether or not they are positively or negatively disposed towards an attitude object and that this only changes if the underlying beliefs change. This unidimensional view of attitudes has been the dominant approach in social psychology (see Eagly and Chaiken 1993).

Recently, however, it has been recognized that attitudes may be multi-dimensional. Thus, rather than attitudes being simply positive *or* negative, individuals can be simultaneously positive *and* negative towards an attitude object. For example, individuals' attitude towards the consumption of junk food may be positive because they like the taste of it, while simultaneously being negative because of the high fat content. This bidimensional view of attitudes is known as **attitudinal ambivalence** (see Thompson *et al.* 1995; Olsen 1999; Conner and Sparks 2001). The idea of attitudinal ambivalence with respect to food choice is particularly appealing, given that food choice has long been associated with ambivalence (Beardsworth 1995) and competing motives (see Herrnstein 1970; Mischel *et al.* 1989). For example, Sparks *et al.* (2001: 56) note that 'people may have mixed feelings about consuming animal products because the sensory appeal of such products may be accompanied by moral concerns with animal welfare issues.' Similarly, the positive evaluations associated with the taste of cream cakes may be experienced simultaneously with negative evaluations concerning weight gain.

As well as capturing potentially conflicting influences on food choice, the consequences of ambivalent attitudes are also important. Given that more ambivalent attitudes capture both positive and negative evaluations of objects, they are likely to be less extreme than less ambivalent (or univalent) attitudes. In other words, they are likely to be weaker than univalent attitudes (see Thompson *et al.* 1995). Of particular relevance to the present discussion, attitudinal ambivalence is likely to moderate the relationship between attitudes and intention/behaviour, such that stronger (i.e. less ambivalent) attitudes are more predictive. A number of recent studies have explored this possibility. For example, Sparks *et al.* (2001) examined ambivalence with respect to eating meat and chocolate and found that greater ambivalence was associated with weaker attitude–intention relationships. Similarly, Povey *et al.* (2001) examined the determinants of eating meat, vegetarian and vegan diets; in each case more ambivalent attitudes were associated with weaker attitude–intention correlations. Thus, Sparks *et al.* (2001) and Povey *et al.* (2001) have found that attitudinal ambivalence undermines the relationship between attitudes and intentions.

Armitage and Conner (2000a: Study 1) replicated these findings in the context of eating a low-fat diet. In addition, they also found that attitudinal ambivalence moderated the attitude–behaviour relationship such that less ambivalent attitudes were more predictive of behaviour three months later. The latter finding is of particular note because it is an example of a study that has simultaneously measured both attitude and intention and found a direct effect of attitude. The implication is that the strong, univalent attitudes by-passed intentions to predict behaviour directly, unmediated by intentions. In a second study, Armitage and Conner (2000a) designed an intervention to change attitudes. The intervention materials were based on the work of Fishbein and Ajzen (1975) and were designed to change beliefs about salient outcomes and the evaluation of those outcomes (see also Ajzen and Fishbein 1980). Examining differences between more and less ambivalent individuals, Armitage and Conner (2000a) found that individuals high in ambivalence were more easily persuaded. Again, this suggests that ambivalent attitudes are weak and therefore more susceptible to a persuasive communication. Thus, research into attitudinal ambivalence suggests that attitudes *can* be predictive of behaviour, but they need to be of a certain strength. In addition, attempts to persuade individuals to change their diet might need to take the strength of attitudes into account.

To date, research on attitudinal ambivalence has focused almost exclusively on what we term *global* ambivalence, or general positive and negative evaluations of behaviour. However, when we are thinking about evaluative conflict with respect to food choice, the conflict between heart and head – or *affect* and *cognition* – is also relevant (Rosenberg and Hovland 1960). Thus, foods can elicit both emotional and cognitive reactions, and attitudinal ambivalence might usefully be extended to incorporate simultaneous affective and cognitive evaluations. For example, a chocolate cake might be simultaneously perceived as enjoyable (positive, affective), beneficial (positive, cognitive), harmful (negative, cognitive) or unpleasant (negative, affective). Given that cognitive outcomes (e.g. health risks, not wasting food) are likely to be more long term than affective outcomes (e.g. pleasure, guilt), it is perhaps unsurprising that health risks are often not predictive of food choice attitudes (e.g. Armitage and Conner 1999a).

Summary and the future of food choice research

We began the chapter by examining sensory and physiological influences on behaviour, arguing that conscious social processes are likely to be more closely related to actual food choice. However, as we have argued towards the end of the chapter, social psychologists have become increasingly interested in affective influences on behaviour. Beyond this, John Bargh (1997: 24) has famously argued that human behaviour is '99 and 44/100% automatic'; that is, social behaviour is principally driven by unconscious processes, rather than the conscious processes (e.g. attitudes) that have traditionally been studied by social psychologists. The evidence for such automaticity of behaviour is powerful, and while it has not yet been examined in relation to food choice, it seems likely that this will be a fruitful area for future research.

By way of an example, Bargh *et al.* (1996: Study 2) surreptitiously exposed (primed) participants to words related to elderly people and compared them with a control group of participants primed with neutral words. Following the priming task, which was introduced as a language test, participants were thanked and allowed to leave. The dependent variable was the speed at which participants walked towards the lift on their way out. Participants primed with the elderly stereotype walked significantly more slowly than individuals in the control group. The influence of automatic processes on behaviour has been demonstrated a number of times, and has been shown to improve cognitive performance (e.g. Dijksterhuis *et al.* 2000) and increase the likelihood of prosocial behaviour (e.g. Macrae and Johnston 1998). It seems likely that similar automatic processes might influence food choices. For example, priming stereotypically thin people (e.g. supermodels) might decrease food consumption; automatic activation of stereotypes of overweight people might increase food consumption. Perhaps more interestingly, given the array of sensory influences on food choice, it is possible that participants might be primed by odour, taste or touch, rather than with manipulations based on linguistic tasks (e.g. the scrambled sentence test).

However, it is unclear what influence these automatic processes will exert outside the laboratory, where priming of a single concept is unlikely to occur. In fact, while these priming effects are robust in laboratory situations, the effects are easily countered by making people self-aware or drawing attention to the prime (e.g. Dijksterhuis *et al.* 2000). Crucially, at least as far as food choice is concerned, Macrae and Johnston (1998) have shown that the introduction of conflicting goals similarly eliminates the effects. Given the breadth of potential goals associated with food choice (e.g. health, self-presentation), it seems unlikely that such effects will be replicated beyond the laboratory. Despite this, research into automatic food choice might provide an opportunity to investigate the relationship between sensory and social influences on food choice.

Beyond the priming studies mentioned above, another way of examining automatic influences on behaviour has been to study the effects of habits on behaviour. Ouellette and Wood (1998) define habits as behaviours that are elicited automatically as a result of situational cues, and demonstrate that past behaviour predicts future behaviour better than intentions in contexts that are conducive to habit formation (i.e. where environments are stable). In terms of food choice, one might therefore expect weekday breakfasts to be better predicted by habit than weekend breakfasts, because the latter are generally less influenced by work patterns. A number of studies of food choice have shown that past behaviour predicts subsequent behaviour, over and above the effects of TPB variables (e.g. Verplanken and Faes 1999; Conner *et al.* 2002). Given that it is impossible truly to manipulate past behaviour (but see Albarracin and Wyer 2000 for a recent attempt to change *perceptions* of past behaviour), the challenge for social psychologists is to identify the variables that explain the relationship between past and future behaviour.

This chapter has examined a range of influences on human food choice as distinct from food preference. Tracing the development of modern behavioural decision-making models, such as the theories of reasoned action and planned behaviour, we discussed the influence of Herrnstein's matching law and optimal foraging theory. Following discussion of the TRA and TPB, we examined where research into these models is going and how we see this research developing in the future. The following chapter considers the contribution social psychologists have made with respect to changing food consumption. Given that the principal motivation behind research into changing food consumption patterns is public health, the next chapter explores ways in which social psychologists have utilized models of health behaviour to inform health interventions.

Notes

1 Note that 'sham feeding' is used as a technique to isolate the effects of CPIR: insulin increases on contact with food, in anticipation of ingestion (see Powley 1977).
2 Ajzen (1991) argues that perceived behavioural control and self-efficacy are synonymous.

Suggested further reading

Birch, L.L. (1999) Development of food preferences, *Annual Review of Nutrition*, 19, 41–62.

A useful review of research that charts the development of food preferences, from genetic predispositions to neophobia, parental feeding practices and learned food preferences.

Eagly, A.H. and Chaiken, S. (1993) *The Psychology of Attitudes*. London: Harcourt Brace Jovanovich.

Nicknamed 'the bible' by researchers in the field, this book provides the most comprehensive review yet of attitude theory and research.

Fishbein, M. and Ajzen, I. (1975) *Belief, Attitude, Intention, and Behavior*. New York: Wiley.

A classic that reviews early research on attitude theory, focusing upon expectancy-value models in particular.

3

Dietary change

General overview

Chapter 2 considered ways in which social psychologists have sought to describe, explain and predict the food choices we make. Implicit within these approaches has been the idea that knowledge of the psychosocial determinants of food choice will facilitate attempts to *change* food choice. The present chapter focuses on social psychological research into dietary change to promote health. This is an important topic for social psychologists and policy-makers alike because common sense and government policy seem to suggest that health is the principal motivating factor in dietary change. Whether in fact this is the case we discuss at the end of the chapter: after all, there are a number of reasons why people might change their diet, many of which we deal with in subsequent chapters. For example, dietary change is implicated in weight-loss attempts, which may or may not be health-motivated (see Chapter 4); dietary intake might change in response to stress (see Chapter 5); and people may manipulate their diet to communicate something about themselves (see Chapter 6).

The present chapter concentrates solely on dietary change to promote health *per se*. First, we review evidence that has looked at the link between dietary intake and health. Second, we examine a number of social psychological models that have been developed to enhance our understanding of dietary change. Third, we examine several approaches to dietary change and consider the extent to which they have adopted social psychological principles to change behaviour. Finally, we summarize the chapter and provide some suggestions for future research.

The link between diet and health

In Chapter 2, we argued that an understanding of the physiology underpinning food choice was essential to developing a model of how we choose certain foods. In this chapter we consider not only how physiology determines the foods we eat, but how the foods we eat exert significant effects on our physiology, which is manifested in our health. There are a number of clear links between diet and health. For example, sugar consumption is linked to dental problems and has been implicated in obesity, and excessive salt intake is related to hypertension and high blood pressure (e.g. Law *et al.* 1991). Of all the potential links between diet and health, though, Western governments have focused attention on the leading causes of death and health expenditure, namely cardiovascular diseases and cancer (e.g. Gardner *et al.* 1996). More specifically, governments have sponsored considerable amounts of research geared towards identifying the key constituents of a 'healthy diet' to reduce the risks of cardiovascular diseases and cancer. As such, compared with work on fat, fibre and fruit and vegetable consumption, there is relatively little research into dietary change with respect to sugar or salt intake because they are regarded as exerting relatively modest effects on health. In the future, there is likely to be more research into broader dietary influences on health, but for the moment, we focus on the two biggest problems: cardiovascular diseases and cancer.

Cardiovascular diseases

Cardiovascular diseases (e.g. strokes, coronary artery disease) are generally thought to be caused by increased levels of cholesterol in the blood. For example, Martin *et al.* (1986) compared men with high and low serum cholesterol levels and found that those in the high cholesterol group were almost three and a half times more likely to die in the next six years than those in the low cholesterol group. Similarly, Stamler *et al.* (1986) followed more than 350,000 adults for six years and found a linear relationship between blood cholesterol level and the incidence of coronary heart disease or stroke. There is now a broad consensus that cholesterol causes cardiovascular disease. Moreover, given that cholesterol is a fat-like substance (although mainly produced in the liver), it was assumed that high fat intake, particularly high saturated fat intake, should be related to levels of cholesterol in the blood. In support of this hypothesis, looking at fat intake, serum cholesterol and incidence of coronary heart disease (CHD), Keys (1980) found correlations in excess of 0.80 between fat and serum cholesterol and between serum cholesterol and incidence of CHD. This would seem to implicate saturated fat as a cause of CHD via increased cholesterol levels. Actually, it has proven difficult to replicate this pattern of findings: for example, Stulb *et al.* (1965) compared the diets of people with high and low blood cholesterol levels and found no differences in dietary intake. As early as 1983, Stallones's review of the literature concluded that there was very little evidence to support a link between fat intake and CHD. The discrepancy between Keys's (1980) data and the studies reviewed by Stallones (1983) is usually attributed to the fact that Keys looked across seven countries, while the studies reviewed by Stallones were conducted within cultures.

There are at least two explanations that are more compelling. First, fat intake has to be lowered considerably before cholesterol levels begin to fall. For example, Temple and Walker (1994) estimate that, in order to achieve significant health benefits, blood cholesterol must be reduced by about 6 per cent. To put this in perspective, clinical trials that have put people on low-fat diets (e.g. 30 per cent of food energy from total fat; 10 per cent of food energy from saturated fat) have produced decrements in serum cholesterol of only 2 per cent (e.g. Ramsay *et al.* 1991). While this is at least partly attributable to poor rates of compliance among those taking part in the trial, it does indicate the difficulty of removing fat from the diet *per se* (see Chapter 4). Related to this, any positive effects are likely to be noticed only in the long term, and Temple (1996) argues that it can take five years for the full benefit to accrue. The implication is that the 'rewards' for reducing fat intake are few and far between and that the health benefits associated with any dietary change are only likely to occur over a period of years, rather than the weeks we often wish for. Thus, whereas fat intake is seen as a major killer on a population level, on an individual level the risks are relatively low. We return to this issue later, in our discussion of the maintenance of dietary change.

The second potential explanation for the weak relationship between fat and cholesterol is that increasing fruit and vegetable intake also reduces cholesterol. For example, Law and Morris (1998) examined the risk of heart disease across groups who differed in the amounts of fruit and vegetables they consumed. The risk of heart disease was between 12 and 19 per cent lower in the highest fruit and vegetable consumption group than in the lowest fruit and vegetable consumption group (Law and Morris 1998). Similarly, evidence suggests that increased consumption of fruit and vegetables confers some protection against strokes. Gillman *et al.* (1995) assessed the fruit and vegetable consumption of 832 men and then observed how many of them had strokes in the next 20 years. Generally speaking, the likelihood of experiencing a stroke decreased as fruit and vegetable consumption increased. More specifically, 19 per cent of the people who ate 0–2 servings[1] per day had a stroke, compared with only 8 per cent of people in the 8–19 servings per day (mean 10 servings per day) group (Gillman *et al.* 1995). Of course, it is possible that people's diets may have changed in the intervening time, so Joshipura *et al.* (1999) took multiple measures of diet over time. They found that eating at least six portions of fruit and vegetables each day reduces the risk of ischaemic stroke by about 30 per cent.

Dietary fibres in general (technically *non-starch polysaccharides*), and in particular those fibres that are soluble in water, are also regarded as a tool for reducing blood cholesterol. Although the independent effects of soluble fibre are hard to tease apart from fruit and vegetable consumption, Brown *et al.*'s (1999) meta-analysis tried to do just this. Brown *et al.* (1999) found that, on average, one gram of soluble fibre reduced blood cholesterol by 0.045 mmol/l (by way of comparison, an apple contains 1 gram of soluble fibre). Thus, it seems that increasing (soluble) fibre intake is likely to confer significant health benefits and could reduce the risk of cardiovascular disease.

Cancer

Diet has also been linked to cancer at a number of sites in the body. In fact, Austoker (1994) estimates that up to 25 per cent of cancer-related deaths are attributable to dietary factors. Austoker (1994) identifies excessive fat intake, lack of fibre and lack of fruit and vegetables as potential causal factors. While the mechanisms are not fully understood, it is thought that diet can influence cancer in three main ways. First, the formation of different cancers might be influenced by the ingestion of carcinogens present in food (e.g. pesticides). Second, the foods ingested may also influence the rate at which cancer cells multiply: for example, the actual chemical structure of certain fatty acids is thought to influence prostaglandins, which in turn are thought to influence cell replication. Third, anti-oxidants contained in fruit and vegetables (e.g. carotenoids, vitamins C and E) have been shown to be protective against some forms of cancer. However, what is clear is that a number of dietary factors are related to cancer.

Excessive fat intake has been linked with increased risk of cancer in the large bowel, lung, endometrium and prostate. For example, Shu *et al.* (1993) reported that high-fat consumers were almost four times more likely to develop endometrium cancer than were low-fat consumers. Similarly, Wynder *et al.* (1987) reported that fat intake was a predictor of lung cancer, even taking smoking into account. However, the link between fat intake and cancer is only correlational: there have been relatively few attempts to manipulate fat intake to prevent cancer, largely due to difficulties in diagnosis (e.g. longer time-lag before symptoms appear).

Fruit and vegetable consumption is more clearly related to cancer. In fact, the amount of fruit and vegetables consumed has been associated with reduced risk of cancer at nearly every site. However, fruit and vegetable consumption seems particularly beneficial in protecting against cancers sited in the oral cavity, larynx, oesophagus and stomach. For example, consumption of citrus fruits and green leafy vegetables has been shown to reduce the risks of oesophageal cancer. Cheng *et al.* (1992) found that those who consumed high levels of fruit and vegetables were between 40 and 60 per cent less likely to be diagnosed with oesophageal cancer. Comparably, Boeing *et al.* (1991) found that people who consumed a lot of fruit and vegetables were between 40 and 30 per cent less at risk of stomach cancer than those who ate few.

Similar findings have been reported with respect to dietary fibre. For example, Jacobs *et al.* (1998) conducted a meta-analysis of the effects of consuming whole-grain products. They found that the vast majority of evidence points to whole grain consumption protecting against various forms of cancer (e.g. gastric, pancreatic, brain). More specifically, their meta-analysis showed that just four (or more) servings of whole grain products per week could reduce the risk of cancer by 40 per cent (Jacobs *et al.* 1998).

Dietary recommendations

The accumulated evidence that supports the link between dietary intake and health has led most governments to draw up guidelines to promote health through eating (e.g. Department of Health and Human Services 1991; Department of Health 1992). But what is a 'healthy diet'? In fact, this is less clear-cut than one might imagine. In considering the evidence above, it seems clear that a low fat, high fruit and vegetable and high fibre diet is 'healthy'. However, it should be noted that these factors are not independent. For example, by increasing fibre intake, one is also less likely to eat food with a high cholesterol content. Similarly, fruit and vegetables are one of the biggest sources of fibre in our diets. In other words, it is difficult to tease apart (for example) the effects of increasing fibre from those of reducing fat intake.

Despite these difficulties, there are several key findings that are likely to remain consistent: a diet that is low fat, high in fruit and vegetables (i.e. at least five portions per day) and high in fibre is likely to confer significant health benefits. It is these facts upon which many governments base their general dietary recommendations. For example, the US government recommends that people should get no more than 30 per cent of their total energy from fat; eat two to four servings of fruit and three to five servings of vegetables; and consume 20–30 grams of dietary fibre every day. In comparison, the UK government recommends that people should get no more than 35 per cent of their total energy from fat; eat 18 grams of dietary fibre (both soluble and insoluble) per day; and eat five portions of fruit and vegetables per day.

There is some evidence to suggest that the message is getting through and that at least some people are eating more healthily. The *Health and Lifestyle Survey* was designed to examine physical and mental well-being in relation to attitudes and lifestyles in a nationally representative sample of the UK. The first *Health and Lifestyle Survey* was conducted in 1984/5 and the second in 1991/2. As part of the analyses of this data set, Prevost *et al.* (1997) were able to track changes in the eating patterns of more than 5,000 people across this seven-year period. Their findings indicated a general reduction in the frequency of consumption of high fat foods (e.g. chips, fried food), but an increase in fast food consumption in younger age groups. Consistent with this, interview studies seem to show that the message about eating fruit and vegetables and avoiding fats is one that is familiar to both healthy eaters and non-healthy eaters alike (e.g. Povey *et al.* 1998). However, despite these apparently encouraging findings, it is clear that the vast majority of people are not adhering to government recommendations (e.g. Kumanyika *et al.* 2000: 44–8). Figure 3.1 shows data adapted from the UK Ministry of

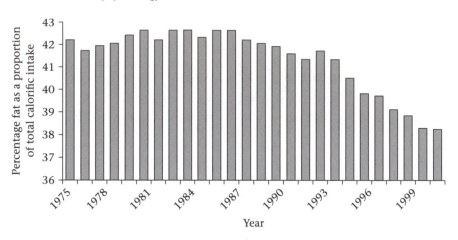

Figure 3.1 Fat as a proportion of total calorific intake in the UK

Agriculture, Fisheries and Food's National Food Survey Branch to show the proportion of total caloric intake derived from fat. Although fat intake has clearly decreased over the years (from 42.3 per cent in 1974 to 38.2 per cent in 2000), average fat consumption in the UK is still some distance from the UK government target of 35 per cent or the US government target of 30 per cent. In response to this, governments have attempted to persuade people to adopt healthier diets of reduced fat and increased fruit, vegetable and fibre consumption.

These dietary recommendations reflect what Glanz (1999) refers to as an 'upstream' intervention: policy-level interventions, which might include economic (e.g. taxation, pricing policy) and legislative (e.g. labelling) strategies. This maps on to what the World Health Organization refers to as 'health public policy', the idea that *all* government policy should take potential public health consequences into account. In referring to **upstream interventions**, Glanz (1999) makes a useful distinction between two other levels: **midstream** and **downstream interventions**. Midstream interventions are classed as those that occur at the level of worksite, schools and even communities. Downstream interventions focus on more intensive interventions, often targeted at 'at-risk' groups (e.g. cancer patients, low socioeconomic status groups). Consistent with the view we expressed in Chapter 2, we believe that social psychologists can make a significant contribution to both understanding and promoting dietary change at each of these levels of intervention. With respect to understanding dietary change, social psychological variables such as beliefs and attitudes (Chapter 2) can be used to evaluate the impact of a range of interventions, whether they be targeted at the individual in a clinic or at a population via television advertising. In fact, as we shall see, social psychological variables are used in order to evaluate the impact of a number of large interventions. Perhaps more importantly, social psychology can be used to promote dietary change, by manipulating key variables. In general, though, it seems that the further 'upstream' one goes, the less effective the intervention and the less the input from social psychologists.

For example, Reger *et al.* (1999) report the effects of a media campaign carried out in the United States. The project was carried out in two communities. In the first, the aim was to encourage people to switch from high-fat to low-fat milk through multimedia presentations (i.e. advertisements on television and radio and in newspapers). In the second community, which was used for comparison, there was no attempt to change milk consumption. The effects of the campaign were analysed by examining sales of low-fat milk one month before and after the campaign. Before the campaign, low-fat milk accounted for 29 per cent of overall milk sales. Immediately after the campaign, low-fat milk sales stood at 46 per cent of total milk sales; six months later low-fat milk sales remained high, at 42 per cent of total milk sales. There were no comparable effects in the no-intervention town. The implication is that the campaign was successful and was effective in reducing the amount of fat consumed in milk.

Another midstream intervention, conducted in Australia, implemented a community-based health promotion programme to complement policy initiatives (Dunt *et al.* 1999). Dunt *et al.* (1999) targeted a community of 50,483 people with two five-week long media (e.g. television, radio) campaigns designed to increase fruit and vegetable consumption ('Fruit 'N' Veg with Every Meal'; Dunt *et al.* 1999: 319) and reduce fat intake ('Flavour without Fat'; Dunt *et al.* 1999: 319). In addition, establishments (e.g. restaurants, cafeterias) that promoted healthy eating were recognized and awarded with plaques; school teachers were provided with teaching materials; school canteen staff were persuaded to offer healthier options; and information kits were given to general practitioners. This first community was then compared with a control community, which received only standard health promotion programmes. Encouragingly, the findings indicated some changes in terms of the perceived interest of the local community in healthy eating. However, the only other significant effects were a decrease in the number of takeaway meals eaten in the experimental community, and Dunt *et al.* (1999: 325) concluded that the interventions were insufficient 'to have any marked impact on either individual dietary behaviour or indeed intention to change dietary behaviour'. Similarly mixed findings have been reported in other midstream interventions (for a review see Glanz 1999).

A related problem concerns the mechanisms for change. For example, while Reger *et al.*'s (1999) intervention clearly changed behaviour, we do not know how the change occurred and therefore cannot isolate the aspects of the campaigns that were effective. Similarly, we are unable to identify whether Reger *et al.* (1999) changed people's beliefs and attitudes, which are likely to drive subsequent healthy eating attempts when the intervention is over. We would argue that these issues can be addressed by reference to social psychological concepts. For example, Dunt *et al.* (1999) did not manage to promote meaningful behaviour change. However, interpreted in terms of the theory of planned behaviour (see Chapter 2), given that they failed to change either intentions or self-efficacy it is perhaps unsurprising that behaviour was not changed.

Understanding dietary change

The contribution of social psychology to the scientific understanding of dietary change has been influential, and examples of the work of social psychologists can be found in many of the leading nutrition journals. Perhaps the key contribution has been the development and application of models of health behaviours to dietary change and subsequent attempts to use that information to promote change. This section examines some of the most popular models of health behaviour: the theory of planned behaviour, the **health belief model**, **protection motivation theory**, **social cognitive theory** and the **transtheoretical model of change**.

Before we discuss these models in detail, it is perhaps useful to draw a distinction between predictive and **explanatory models** (Sutton 1998). *Predictive models* identify key variables that are correlated with people's health behaviour; this information can be used to identify, with some level of certainty, the people who are likely to (for example) require attention from a dietician. By way of an example, given that attitudes are predictive of food choice (see Chapter 2), one could identify all the people with negative attitudes and engage them in a dietary education programme. *Explanatory models* are distinct from predictive models insofar as the key variables are held to play a causal role in determining behaviour. To take our people with negative attitudes towards eating a low-fat diet again, if attitudes are explanatory variables, we would deliberately try to change their attitudes, in the knowledge that any shift in attitude should produce a corresponding shift in behaviour. This distinction between predictive and explanatory is important because explanatory variables are necessarily predictive, whereas predictive variables are not necessarily explanatory (Sutton 1998). Consistent with this distinction, researchers have tended to use models of health behaviour either to predict dietary change or to explain dietary change. In other words, models of health behaviour have been used to evaluate the effectiveness of dietary change interventions (i.e. in a predictive manner) and to change health behaviour by changing specific variables.

This section reviews work on the theory of planned behaviour, the health belief model, protection motivation theory, social cognitive theory and the transtheoretical model. A brief description of each model is presented, followed by a brief review of ways in which the model has been used in dietary change. Generally, there are two ways in which such models are used. First, key variables are taken from the models and are used to predict change by evaluating the effectiveness of a health campaign (e.g. Dunt *et al.* 1999). Second, these models can be used to explain dietary change by manipulating specific variables to promote actual dietary change.

Theory of planned behaviour

We examined the theory of planned behaviour (TPB) (Ajzen 1991, 1998) in some depth in Chapter 2. Briefly, the model taps attitudinal, social and motivational (i.e. intentions and self-efficacy) influences on behaviour, and has been researched extensively as a model of food choice (see Chapter 2). In addition, a number of researchers have used the model to examine dietary change (see also Chapter 4 on dietary change in relation to weight loss). Consistent with the distinction between prediction and explanation of behaviour, the TPB has been used both to predict dietary change and to promote dietary change.

Measures from the TPB have been used to predict dietary change, typically by examining differences in TPB variables following the administration of a dietary intervention. For example, Anderson *et al.* (1998) tested 'Take Five', a nutrition education package designed to increase fruit and vegetable consumption, using measures from the TPB. They found that a number of beliefs changed during the intervention period, notably about the link between diet and cancer and vegetables being a good source of protein (see Anderson *et al.* 1998). Similarly, Kristal *et al.* (2000) measured beliefs, attitudes and behavioural intention ('motivation') before and after an intervention designed to promote fruit and vegetable consumption and reduce fat intake. Kristal *et al.* (2000) reported significant differences in these variables, as well as evidence to suggest that their sample were eating more healthily.

Fewer studies have used the TPB to promote dietary change, although Ajzen and Fishbein (1980) have suggested a number of ways in which TPB-related models (e.g. the earlier theory of reasoned action) can be used to change behavioural intentions and behaviour. Their approach focuses on the targeting of underlying beliefs. As we described in Chapter 2, attitudes, subjective norms and perceived behavioural control are held to be determined by salient behavioural, normative and control beliefs, respectively (Ajzen 1991). Ajzen and Fishbein (1980) argue that changing these underlying beliefs should bring about long-lasting change in (for example) attitudes, intentions and behaviour.

Generally speaking, there are two stages involved in using the TPB to develop an intervention. First, it is important to determine which variables should be targeted: clearly, it would be counter-productive to target variables that did not account for variance in behavioural intention or behaviour. Second, the message content must be identified. This is done either by identifying new salient beliefs that the recipient has not yet heard of or by targeting existing salient beliefs. Given that the focus of the present chapter is on dietary change, it seems unlikely that anyone would be able to generate new beliefs about the foods that people are currently eating. The focus of any dietary change study would therefore be on changing existing salient beliefs.

Even though Ajzen and Fishbein's (1980) recommendations were published more than two decades ago, attempts to utilize the TPB to design interventions have been few and far between. Those studies that have been conducted have met with mixed results and were not designed to promote dietary change (see Armitage and Conner 2002 for a review). There are a number of reasons why there have been few attempts to study the TPB systematically as a model of dietary change, of which four seem to be the most compelling. First, as we have outlined above, developing an intervention based on the TPB is likely to be very expensive and time-consuming. In contrast, it is far cheaper (and easier) to examine the correlates of behaviour, before going on to speculate that such correlates might be useful in changing behaviour.

The second potential barrier to developing interventions based on the TPB is actually more plausible. Given that past experience has been shown to strengthen attitudes, for a habitual behaviour like food choice attitudes are likely to be very strong and therefore more difficult to change. If this is the case, the only way to change food choice attitudes would be to try to weaken existing attitudes, or target individuals whose attitudes are weak to begin with. As far as we are aware, no one has attempted the former with respect to dietary change, but several studies have attempted to take advantage of existing weak attitudes to target them with an intervention. For example, Armitage and Conner (2000a: Study 2) developed a health message that was designed to change people's behavioural beliefs with respect to eating a low-fat diet (i.e. the perceived likelihood of outcomes occurring and the evaluation of those outcomes; see Chapter 2). Following piloting, salient behavioural beliefs were identified that discriminated those who intended to eat a low-fat diet from those who did not, and a persuasive message designed to target those beliefs was developed. The effects of the message were clear: people with weaker (i.e. more ambivalent) attitudes were more persuaded to eat a low-fat diet than people with stronger (i.e. less ambivalent) attitudes. Thus, taking attitude strength into account when targeting messages might enhance the impact of such persuasive messages.

Third, within the TPB, attitude and subjective norms are actually relatively weak predictors of behaviour. While attitude is typically the strongest predictor of intention, intention is usually the strongest predictor of behaviour: the effects of attitudes are usually indirect and mediated through behavioural intentions (but see Armitage and Conner 2000a: Study 1). The implication is that the most efficient way to change behaviour would be to target intentions directly. In fact, Verplanken and Faes (1999) have done just this. As we described in Chapter 2, Verplanken and Faes (1999) actually increased levels of healthy eating by asking their participants to form specific plans (*implementation intentions*) about when and how to eat healthily. Perceived behavioural control is also a direct predictor of behaviour within the TPB, and so provides

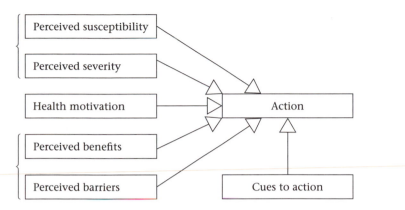

Figure 3.2 The health belief model

another potential route to dietary change. However, given that Ajzen (1998) regards perceived behavioural control and self-efficacy as being synonymous, we will return to this issue later.

Fourth, the TPB was designed as a model of general social behaviour, rather than as a model of health behaviour or health behaviour change. Potentially, the TPB might be considered far removed from the field of dietary change, and researchers have therefore adopted models developed specifically to address health behaviour and to study dietary change. The following section reviews a number of key models of health behaviour and examines ways in which they have been used to inform interventions designed to promote dietary change.

Health belief model

The health belief model (HBM) is actually one of the oldest models of health behaviour. Work on it began by observing that several social groups were underrepresented in screening programmes, notably men and people of lower socioeconomic status. Noting that sociodemographic variables such as gender and social class were unlikely to determine behaviour *per se*, and that such variables are not readily amenable to change, researchers began to identify psychosocial variables that would explain the relationship between social demography and behaviour. According to the HBM (Rosenstock 1974; Janz and Becker 1984), there are six determinants of health behaviour: **perceived susceptibility, perceived severity, perceived benefits, perceived barriers, health motivation** and **cues to action** (see Figure 3.2). Thus, the effects of sociodemographic variables on behaviour are explained in terms of differences in each of these variables (e.g. men may feel less susceptible to disease).

Perceived susceptibility and perceived severity are often paired together to give an index of **perceived threat**. Thus (for example), people who believe they are relatively susceptible to CHD and perceive CHD as being severe are more likely to perceive a threat to themselves and are more likely to act to reduce this threat (e.g. by reducing cholesterol). In addition, people are held to make judgements about the means they will use to actually achieve their goal. For example, one way of reducing one's risk of CHD is by lowering blood cholesterol, but people are only likely to follow this course of action if they believe that there are benefits in doing this and if they perceive few barriers. Thus, individuals are more likely to reduce saturated fat if they: (a) believe it will confer personal benefits (e.g. reduce their risk of CHD); and (b) believe there are relatively few barriers (e.g. they know about what to eat to reduce their cholesterol). Beyond this, individuals are more likely to act if they are motivated to look after their health ('health motivation') and if there are specific cues to action (e.g. pains in the chest, health promotion campaign).

There have been a number of applications of the HBM to the study of food choice and dietary change. For example, Sapp and Jensen (1998) found that the HBM was a good predictor of health-related food choice in a nationally representative sample of 1,502 individuals, with the benefits ('importance of diet') being an especially important predictor of a number of diet-related indices. Similarly, Schafer et al. (1995) reported that the HBM was a good predictor of fat intake, accounting for almost 30 per cent of the variance in behaviour, and found that their sample were most likely to be motivated by the perceived costs of eating a healthier diet.

Chew et al. (1998) used the HBM to evaluate the impact of a one-hour television programme about diet and nutrition. Before the programme was broadcast, Chew et al. (1998) contacted 997 people and measured components of the HBM as well as their dietary intake. After broadcast, the participants were contacted and their health beliefs and behaviour were assessed. Chew et al. (1998) reported significant improvements in several HBM constructs: response efficacy (i.e. more perceived benefits, less perceived barriers), health motivation, salience ('concern about food and fitness') and cues to action ('confidence in information'). Perhaps more importantly, people who had seen the programme also reported eating more healthily than before. Unfortunately, Chew et al. (1998) decided to discard the 581 people who had not watched the programme and instead focused their analyses on those ($n = 416$) who had viewed the programme. Thus, it is not clear whether the effects are attributable to the programme or not.

The HBM provides a summary of variables that are assumed to be important in determining health behaviour. However, we were unable to locate any studies that tested interventions designed to manipulate HBM variables to influence diet per se. Having said that, a number of researchers have used the HBM as a broad framework around which to design interventions, including those designed to enhance self-efficacy and provide people with personal risk information, which we review below. Moreover, the HBM provides a way of understanding the effects of health promotion campaigns that work through the media (e.g. Reger *et al.* 1999): such campaigns may simply trigger cues to action. Unfortunately, quite what constitutes a 'cue to action' is under debate and several commentators have identified other potential problems with the HBM in general, which we examine below.

First, in general the six HBM components are regarded as independent predictors of behaviour. However, implicit in the conceptualization of the HBM are interactive effects between some of the variables (see Sheeran and Abraham 1996). For example, the combination of perceived susceptibility and perceived severity are regarded as producing a measure of perceived threat; the combination of perceived benefits and perceived barriers provides a measure of response efficacy (i.e. is this course of action going to benefit me?). At a higher level, do people engage in health behaviours purely because of a threat, without taking account of the potential benefits or barriers? In fact, there is surprisingly little work that has investigated any of these issues.

Second, critics of the HBM have argued that the components are not consistently operationalized because they are not clearly defined. For example, Sapp and Jensen (1998: 240) operationalized cues to action as 'whether the respondent was on any type of special diet', whereas others have operation-alized them as 'respondents' confidence in assessing the quality of dietary information (confidence in information) and the need for reliable informa-tion' (Chew *et al.* 1998: 235). By the same token, what *is* a 'cue to action'? A cue to action might include physical symptoms associated with (for example) CHD or diabetes, which might otherwise be regarded as a threat (i.e. increasing perceived susceptibility or perceived severity). Alternatively, a cue to action may be a persuasive message that influences one's perceived response efficacy.

Third, evidence for predictive validity is only equivocal. For example, Harrison *et al.*'s (1992) meta-analysis of the HBM did not include cues to action or health motivation because of the dearth of studies measuring these constructs. Moreover, although all correlations between the HBM and beha-viour were significant, the effect sizes were small (all $r < 0.21$; see Sheeran and Abraham 1996). Consistent with this, studies that have directly compared the HBM with other models (e.g. theory of planned behaviour) have found that the HBM is a weaker predictor of behaviour (e.g. Conner and Norman 1994). More recent studies have therefore focused on protection motivation theory – a model developed out of the HBM.

Protection motivation theory

Rogers's (1983) protection motivation theory (PMT) is regarded as an extension of the HBM and they share a number of key variables in common (see Figure 3.3). However, the roots of the model can be found in work on **fear appeals**, the idea that generating fear in people should make them act to protect themselves (Rogers 1983). Protection motivation theory identifies a number of key variables that are held to mediate the effects of fear appeals on self-protective behaviour. Thus, within PMT, health behaviour is ultimately

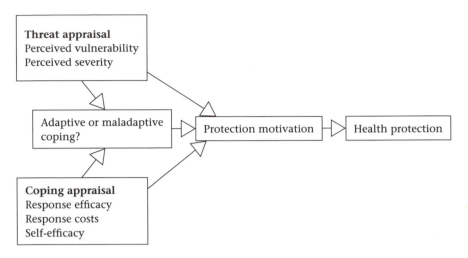

Figure 3.3   Protection motivation theory

determined by one's motivation to protect oneself (**protection motivation**). In turn, protection motivation is determined by an appraisal of the threat itself and ways in which one might respond to that threat. Comparable with the HBM, threat appraisal is determined by **perceived vulnerability** and perceived severity. Thus, if you perceive yourself as being vulnerable to (for example) CHD and you believe CHD is severe, the motivation to protect yourself is increased. **Threat appraisal** therefore takes into account one's current behaviour and evaluates whether there is sufficient threat to act. If one feels sufficient threat, the process of **coping appraisal** determines whether one is motivated to protect oneself. Coping appraisal is based on three types of information: the perceived usefulness of the responses (**response efficacy**), the costs and benefits associated with the response (**response cost**) and confidence in one's own ability to perform the behaviour (**self-efficacy**). For example, reducing saturated fat intake may be perceived to be a useful response to the threat of CHD, but protection motivation might actually be weak because there are more costs than benefits or because self-efficacy is low.

Despite the fact that PMT has been the subject of a number of empirical investigations (for recent reviews see Boer and Seydel 1996; Floyd *et al.* 2000; Milne *et al.* 2000), we were able to locate just two studies that had fully operationalized the model in the domain of dietary change. Plotnikoff and Higginbotham (1995) used PMT to predict intentions and behaviour with respect to eating a low-fat diet. Response efficacy and self-efficacy were the dominant predictors of intention, suggesting that if people are confident that a low-fat diet reduces cholesterol and are confident in their own ability to eat a low-fat diet, they are more likely to intend to do so. More importantly, intention and self-efficacy were significant predictors of behaviour, accounting for 39 per cent of the variance. Interestingly, Plotnikoff and Higginbotham (1995) also included a measure of fear of CHD, which was not directly predictive of behaviour, but influenced perceived vulnerability, perceived severity and response efficacy.

A more direct test of the latter finding is provided by Wurtele (1988), who reports a study designed to inform female students about the risks of osteoporosis and persuade them to increase their calcium intake as a preventive measure. Wurtele's (1988) paper reports data on three outcome measures (taking calcium supplements, eating a calcium-rich diet and taking a free calcium supplement), but in keeping with the rest of the chapter, we will focus on the findings relating to eating a calcium-rich diet. Wurtele (1988) gave participants information that was designed to induce high (or low) perceived vulnerability and high (or low) response efficacy. Findings indicated that the vulnerability manipulation significantly increased perceived vulnerability, intentions and behaviour (the latter measured two weeks later). The response efficacy manipulation actually increased participants' response efficacy, but the effects did not carry forward to intentions or actual consumption of a calcium-rich diet. The second part of Wurtele's (1988) analyses used PMT to predict intention and behaviour. Together, perceived vulnerability and response efficacy predicted intentions to eat a calcium-rich diet; intention alone accounted for 17 per cent of the variance in dietary intake.

Even though we were only able to identify two studies that tested PMT specifically in relation to dietary change, both Wurtele (1988) and Plotkinoff and Higginbotham (1995) provide evidence to support the predictive validity of PMT. The implication is that increasing people's perceived vulnerability to disease should increase the likelihood of people changing their diet. In fact, as we shall see below, recent research that has provided people with personal dietary feedback has proven very successful in changing people's diets, even over long periods of time.

However, despite broad empirical support for the conceptualization of PMT, some of the criticisms attached to the HBM can equally be applied to PMT (see above). Similarly, the predictive validity of its unique components is modest. For example, vulnerability to disease could be interpreted as the perceived likelihood of a certain outcome occurring (i.e. a behavioural belief; see Chapter 2). Perhaps more importantly, as acknowledged by both Wurtele (1988) and Plotnikoff and Higginbotham (1995), the proximal determinants of behaviour in both studies (i.e. intention and self-efficacy) are actually more closely associated with the theory of planned behaviour (see Ajzen 1991).

Social cognitive theory

Unlike the HBM or PMT, Bandura's (1986, 1997) social cognitive theory (SCT) is probably best known for a single construct: self-efficacy. Self-efficacy relates to confidence in one's own ability to carry out a particular behaviour (Bandura 1986, 1997), and can also be found in PMT and the TPB (see Ajzen

1998). The idea is that the more confident you are in your own ability to eat a healthy diet, the more likely you are to do so. In addition to self-efficacy, SCT also includes measures of outcome expectancies, which are somewhat similar to the behavioural beliefs that underpin the theories of reasoned action and planned behaviour (see Chapter 2). What is different about outcome expectancies in Bandura's (1986) model is that he makes a distinction between situation-outcome and action-outcome expectancies and regards them as determinants of behaviour. **Situation-outcome expectancies** are based on the perception that some consequences are determined by the environment and are thus divorced from personal control. **Action-outcome expectancies** are likewise related to the belief that one's actions are instrumental to a particular outcome. SCT therefore predicts that behaviours are performed if one perceives control over the outcome, few external barriers and confidence in one's own ability. For example, you are more likely to increase fibre consumption if you believe that you are able to eat more fibre, that your situation is likely to facilitate this and that you are confident you will be able to resist high-fat foods.

SCT has been shown to be a useful predictor of a variety of health behaviours and behavioural intentions (see Schwarzer and Fuchs 1996 for a review). However, the full model has rarely been applied to dietary change, with a number of researchers focusing on the self-efficacy construct alone. Some notable exceptions include Sheeshka *et al.* (1993), who found that both self-efficacy and outcome expectancies predicted intentions to eat healthily (e.g. reduce the amount of butter used, eat at least three servings of vegetables every day). Resnicow *et al.* (1997) examined the predictive validity of SCT with respect to the fruit and vegetable intake of children. Resnicow *et al.* (1997) found that the outcome expectancy (but not self-efficacy) component was predictive of their behaviour across a seven-day period. Similarly, Schwarzer and Fuchs (1996) studied 800 people and their eating behaviour across a six-month time period, and found that positive outcome expectancies, self-efficacy and behavioural intentions were all predictive of behaviour, accounting for 20–21 per cent of the variance.

Finally, in a recent extension of SCT, Schwarzer and Renner (2000) distinguished between action self-efficacy and coping self-efficacy. They defined action self-efficacy as confidence in one's ability to perform the behaviour (eat a low-fat, high-fibre diet in this study) and coping self-efficacy as confidence in one's ability to maintain that behaviour. Consistent with their hypotheses, Schwarzer and Renner (2000) found that action self-efficacy, outcome expectancies and perceived risk were predictive of intentions and coping self-efficacy, but that intentions and coping self-efficacy were predictive of subsequent behaviour.

Studies that have utilized SCT as a basis for designing interventions have focused almost exclusively on self-efficacy and are mainly related to weight control. For example, as part of a larger study, Shannon *et al.* (1990) assessed 180 clerical assistants in terms of self-efficacy with respect to choosing appropriate foods before and after they embarked upon a ten-week weight-loss course. The data show that the course significantly increased self-efficacy and significantly reduced fat intake, calorific intake and body weight. Although the findings must be interpreted with some caution because there was no control group and there was only an indirect measure of *dietary* change, the implication is that enhancing self-efficacy is likely to change food choice and thereby exert effects on weight loss (see Chapter 4 for further examples).

Howard-Pitney *et al.* (1997) report a large-scale intervention that drew upon SCT by providing food tasting, demonstrations, active learning and skills teaching, precisely the kind of features that one might expect to enhance self-efficacy (see below; see also Bandura 1986). In other words, they not only showed their participants the outcomes of eating healthy foods, they provided role models, mastery experiences and persuasive messages. More importantly, their intervention produced 2.3 per cent greater reduction in the proportion of calories derived from fat than the control condition. Those studies that have used self-efficacy alone to promote dietary change are discussed in the following section.

Transtheoretical model of change

In contrast with the models reviewed thus far, Prochaska and DiClemente's (1983, 1984) transtheoretical model (TTM) developed from a 'bottom-up' perspective. That is, rather than hypothesizing about the kind of influences that might be important influences on behaviour change, Prochaska and DiClemente built their model on observations of psychotherapy sessions (see Prochaska 1979). Central to their model is the idea that people pass through similar **stages of change** regardless of the type of therapy or the sort of problem they may have. The implication is that no matter what kind of behaviour is under consideration, individuals should move through a series of distinguishable stages: **precontemplation, contemplation, preparation, action** and **maintenance** (see Figure 3.4).

The first stage, the *precontemplation* stage, includes individuals who have no intention to change their behaviour in the foreseeable future. Thus, precontemplators are assumed to be unaware or underaware that their current behaviour constitutes a problem. The *contemplation* stage is characterized by people who are thinking about making a change in the next six months, but have yet to take any kind of action. *Preparation* is the third stage, where individuals intend to take action and have gone some way towards taking this action. For example, people might start to purchase low-fat spreads as opposed to butter. Once individuals have successfully managed to perform the behaviour in question, they are labelled as being in the *action* stage. Individuals are regarded as being in the final (*maintenance*) stage once they have been performing the behaviour in question for six months or more.

The stages of change have been applied to a number of health behaviours (e.g. Sutton 2000) and, to a lesser extent, food choice. de Graaf *et al.* (1997)

measured the stages of change of a nationally representative sample of 14,331 members of the European Union. The target behaviour was eating a healthier diet. de Graaf *et al.* (1997) found that across all European Union countries, 52 per cent of participants regarded themselves as precontemplators, compared with 2 per cent who regarded themselves as contemplators, 1 per cent in the preparation stages, 7 per cent in the action stage and 31 per cent in the maintenance stage. Notably, individuals from Germany and those in Mediterranean countries were more likely to be precontemplators (55–64 per cent) than those in Scandinavian countries (20–38 per cent). These findings are unusual: one would normally expect a more even spread of participants across the stages. For example, Armitage and Conner (2001a) examined the stages of change for consuming a low-fat diet: 9 per cent of their sample were in precontemplation, 12 per cent in contemplation, 39 per cent in preparation, 11 per cent in action and 29 per cent in maintenance (cf. Laforge *et al.* 1999). One explanation for the discrepancy between these findings is that de Graaf *et al.* (1997) asked their participants about *healthier* eating. Potentially, this is ambiguous: someone who is already eating healthily and is therefore not considering *healthier* eating would be classified as a precontemplator in de Graaf *et al.*'s study. Consistent with this view, closer examination of de Graaf *et al.*'s figures reveals that 77 per cent of their precontemplators regarded themselves as 'already healthy' eaters. More convincing still are studies that examine actual dietary consumption across the stages of change. Armitage and Conner (2001a) examined levels of fat intake across the five stages of change and found that people in the earlier stages (e.g. precontemplation, contemplation) were consuming more fat than individuals in the later stages (e.g. action, maintenance).

The stages of change component is undoubtedly the most widely researched part of the TTM, although Prochaska and DiClemente have identified two further groups of variables, known as the **processes of change** and the *mediators of change*. The processes of change are ten strategies that individuals use to move themselves between stages (see Marcus *et al.* 1992). These processes of change are divided into experiential and behavioural processes. Broadly speaking, the **experiential processes** represent ways in which people progress through the stages of change, while the **behavioural processes** are associated with preventing relapse (e.g. Marcus *et al.* 1992; Prochaska *et al.* 1994a).

The five experiential processes are: **consciousness raising, dramatic relief, environmental re-evaluation, self-re-evaluation** and **social liberation.** Consciousness raising involves obtaining new information about a particular health issue (e.g. by collecting information about levels of dietary fat). Dramatic relief is the emotional experience of change, such as unhappiness associated with not eating cream cakes when one is on a low-fat diet. Environmental re-evaluation involves the identification of social and physical influences on one's behaviour; for example, by identifying situations that might lead to eating fatty foods. Self-re-evaluation involves the examination of one's beliefs and attitudes about eating healthily (e.g. a low-fat diet can be tasty). Social liberation is concerned with changes in one's social identity such that it is possible to see one's self as (for example) a healthy eater.

Five behavioural processes are also elucidated: **counter-conditioning, helping relationships, reinforcement management, self-liberation** and **stimulus control**. *Counter-conditioning* involves replacing the problem behaviour with alternative behaviours (e.g. choosing low-fat options). *Helping relationships* tap social support and the way in which people use their relationships with others to help them change their diet (e.g. by forming pacts with friends to avoid eating fast food). *Reinforcement management* involves re-evaluating the way in which food is used as a reward or punishment. *Self-liberation* taps people's commitment to change. *Stimulus control* involves the monitoring of potential triggers to the behaviour (e.g. avoiding fast food while passing an outlet). The implication is that each of these processes could be used to guide people who want to change their diet.

As far as we are aware, no studies have yet examined the processes of change with respect to dietary change and this is an avenue for further research. Instead, researchers have tended to focus on the mediators of change, namely *self-efficacy* and *decisional balance*. This is because the processes of change are held to exert their influence on behaviour via self-efficacy and **decisional balance**. In other words, self-efficacy and decisional balance mediate the effects of the processes of change on behaviour and can therefore be regarded as predictors of stage transitions. We encountered self-efficacy above (see also Bandura 1997). Decisional balance, on the other hand, is based on work by Janis and Mann (1977) and is concerned with the pros and cons that people generate when considering whether or not to perform a particular behaviour. The idea is that once the number of pros outweigh the number of cons, one is more likely to act in a 'pro' direction. Interestingly, the ideas of balancing pros and cons overlaps to some extent with the idea of attitudinal ambivalence, introduced in Chapter 2. Attitudinal ambivalence is concerned with the simultaneous possession of both positive and negative thoughts/feelings about a particular object. Extrapolating the ideas of decisional balance on to those of attitudinal ambivalence, one might therefore expect people to be less ambivalent about dietary change in the precontemplation and maintenance stages than in the contemplation, preparation and action stages. In fact, a recent study by Armitage *et al.* (2002) produced just such a pattern of findings in relation to eating a low-fat diet and consuming five portions of fruit and vegetables per day.

There is ample support for the effects of self-efficacy and decisional balance across the stages of change. For example, Prochaska *et al.* (1994b) examined the stages of change in conjunction with decisional balance for reducing fat intake. They found that the pros of reducing fat intake *increased*, while the cons of reducing fat intake *decreased* across the stages of change. The implication is that at some point between precontemplation and action, the number of pros outweighs the number of cons and people decide to eat more healthily

Stages of change	Precontemplation		Contemplation			Preparation			Action			Maintenance	
Definition	'I currently do not eat a healthy diet and I am not thinking about starting.'		'I currently do not eat a healthy diet but I am thinking about starting.'			'I currently eat a healthy diet but not on a regular basis.'			'I currently eat a healthy diet but I have only begun to do so in the last six months.'			'I currently eat a healthy diet and I have done so for longer than six months.'	
Movement	0	+	–	0	+	–	0	+	–	0	+	–	0
Group number	1	2	3	4	5	6	7	8	9	10	11	12	13
No. of participants	30	16	4	16	40	18	131	43	23	11	22	26	119

–, relapse; 0, static; +, progress.

Figure 3.4 The stages of change and 13 possible 'changes of stage'

Source: adapted from Armitage et al. 2002.

(Prochaska *et al.* 1994b). Comparably, Armitage and Arden (2002) found that self-efficacy for eating a low-fat diet increased in a linear fashion across the stages of change. In other words, lower self-efficacy was perceived in the pre-contemplation stage relative to the contemplation stage; in the contemplation stage relative to the preparation stage; and so on.

The implication is that increasing feelings of self-efficacy or the number of pros is likely to promote dietary change. However, each of these studies is cross-sectional and actually tells us relatively little about the variables that are likely to move people from one stage to the next (see Sutton 2000). Moreover, we already know that promoting self-efficacy or making people's thoughts more positive is likely to promote dietary change (Shannon *et al.* 1990; Armitage and Conner 2000a), so what are the stages of change truly contributing to our knowledge? One potential contribution that the TTM could make would be to assist in our understanding of dynamic change, or *changes in stage* across time.

Very few studies have tried to investigate stage transitions in the context of the TTM and dietary change, and often these have collapsed across the stages of change in order to facilitate data analysis (e.g. Kristal *et al.* 2000: 114–15). One exception is a recent study by Armitage *et al.* (2002), who set out to examine transitions between the stages of change across a period of eight months. More specifically, they wanted to see if it was possible to predict changes in stage, using variables derived from the theory of planned behaviour.[2] Participants were divided into 13 groups (see Figure 3.4) according to which stage of change they were in, and whether they relapsed (i.e. moved to an earlier stage), remained static or progressed (i.e. moved to a subsequent stage). In fact, across the five-month time period, there were relatively few changes of stage: more than 60 per cent of participants remained in their original stage, with 14 per cent relapsing and 24 per cent progressing. Analyses revealed that TPB variables were predictive of movements between most of the stages of change. For example, perceived behavioural control (i.e. self-efficacy; see Ajzen 1998) predicted progression from both the contemplation and action stages. Thus, in general, Armitage *et al.*'s (2002) data provide support for the TTM.

The one exception to this pattern of findings was the progression from preparation to action (i.e. movement between group numbers 8 and 9 in Figure 3.4). However, in some senses, the progression from preparation to action is *the* crucial stage transition because it marks the translation from mental preparedness to actual action. People in the preparation stage are making only half-hearted attempts at the target behaviour (e.g. by occasionally purchasing foods that are lower in fat) in comparison with those in the action or maintenance stage, who have been eating healthily for some time. The inability to predict this stage transition is therefore problematic. In fact, we regard this transition between cognition and action as being formally equivalent to the 'intention–behaviour gap' discussed towards the end of Chapter 2 (e.g. Kuhl 1985; Gollwitzer 1993; Sheeran 2002). There, we suggested that practical (volitional) strategies such as *implementation intentions* would be important in ensuring that cognitions are translated into action. To date, implementation intentions have not been tested in conjunction with the TTM. However, accumulated evidence suggests that they might facilitate dietary change (e.g. Verplanken and Faes 1999; for a review see Sheeran 2002). Moreover, given that implementation intention interventions are typically formed on a person-by-person basis, the effects might mirror those found for the **tailored interventions** that are reviewed in the following section. In general, further research, particularly research adopting prospective designs, is required.

The stages of change component of the TTM has successfully discriminated five potential groups (precontemplation, contemplation, preparation, action, maintenance) at which interventions could be targeted. Therefore, one of the most promising avenues for research into the TTM is to investigate the effects of stage-matched **targeted interventions**. As with studies of the TTM in general, dietary change has not been a focus of research attention, although there have been a number of promising studies. For example, Steptoe *et al.* (1999) randomized people to either a control or an intervention condition. Participants in the intervention condition received counselling that was designed to change attitudes and encourage participants to develop plans to change, depending on their stage of change. In other words, the study provided stage-matched interventions. Steptoe *et al.*'s (1999) findings indicated that fat intake was reduced in the intervention group, even over a 12-month period, suggesting that stage-matched interventions might be a useful tool in promoting dietary change. However, as with all tailored interventions (see below), the findings should be interpreted with some caution: Steptoe *et al.*'s (1999) intervention was not targeted solely at diet (it included exercise and cigarette smoking) and included only high-risk participants. Moreover, from a theoretical viewpoint, a more powerful test of the TTM would be to demonstrate that stage-matched interventions are better at changing people's diet than are stage-*mis*matched interventions (see Weinstein *et al.* 1998 for discussion of this and related issues). Despite these notes of caution, we regard work of the kind carried out by Steptoe and colleagues as an essential step in the process of understanding dietary change.

Steptoe *et al.*'s (1999) use of the TTM to target interventions reflects a more general trend of targeting and tailoring interventions, which has almost exclusively been developed in the field of dietary change. We examine some of this work in the following section.

Targeting and tailoring interventions

Before considering ways in which researchers have sought to maximize the impact of dietary interventions through targeting and tailoring, we ought to explain what we mean by targeting and tailoring. Kreuter and Skinner (2000) regard the distinction between targeting and tailoring as important because the two terms have often been used interchangeably. On the one hand, *targeted* interventions are regarded as those that have been designed 'for a defined population subgroup that takes into account characteristics shared by the subgroup's members' (Kreuter and Skinner 2000: 1). In contrast, tailored interventions are '*intended to reach one specific person*, based on characteristics unique to that person . . . *derived from an individual assessment*' (Kreuter and Skinner 2000: 1; emphasis in original). Thus, any attempt to develop interventions on the basis of the five stages of change would be regarded as a targeted intervention, whereas providing people with personalized feedback would be regarded as a tailored intervention. Historically, tailored dietary interventions have been intensive, expensive and only aimed at high-risk individuals (e.g. those with high blood pressure). In general, these have been successful in changing people's diets (e.g. Brunner *et al.* 1997). In contrast, attempts to change the diet of the general population have generally been cheaper, but less intensive and less successful (e.g. Maccoby *et al.* 1977; Family Heart Study Group 1994; OXCHECK Study Group 1994; Dunt *et al.* 1999).

A relatively early example is provided by Campbell *et al.* (1994), who compared the effectiveness of an intervention tailored by the stage of change, behaviour, beliefs and attitudes of participants, with a control condition. The tailored messages seemed to be most effective at reducing total and saturated fat intake, but did not increase fruit and vegetable consumption. In addition, people in the tailored condition were more likely both to remember receiving the message and to report reading it (Campbell *et al.* 1994). Thus, there seems to be some evidence to suggest that stage-matched interventions are more likely to improve dietary intake than are non-stage matched interventions. Moreover, it is perhaps unsurprising that tailoring is more effective at reducing fat intake than increasing fruit and vegetable consumption, given that fat is often 'hidden' in food.

There have now been several interventions, which, like Campbell *et al.* (1994), have used computer programs to analyse participants' responses and tailor interventions to suit them. Although not necessarily using concepts from the TTM, these studies have generally improved dietary intake. Based on their review of eight such studies, Brug *et al.* (1999) conclude that computer-tailored interventions exert significant effects on dietary change. In particular, people are more likely to attend to, remember and find tailored information more personally relevant than standard information. In addition, such information is more likely to motivate people to change their diet (see Brug *et al.* 1999). Beyond this, it seems that it is not always necessary to target specific beliefs or attitudes. For example, Beresford *et al.* (1997) found that simply providing participants with a self-help manual, a brief motivational message from their physician and a reminder letter two weeks later improved people's diets. Those in the intervention group significantly increased their fibre consumption and decreased their fat consumption compared with the no-treatment controls. Moreover, the effects remained when reassessed 12 months later.

However, the problem with tailoring studies and other 'downstream' interventions (see Glanz 1999) is that, inevitably, the experimental materials exert demands on people that are often not controlled for. In other words, the tailored message is likely to be longer, more detailed and more intensive than the materials (if any) given to the comparison group. For example, Beresford *et al.* (1997) provided participants in the intervention group with not only a self-help manual but a motivational message from their physician and a reminder letter. Thus, which is the effective part of the intervention: the leaflet, the physician's message, the reminder or some combination of the three? In a related study, Campbell and colleagues (1994: 787) concede that 'The tailored messages were personalised and provided more information than did the non-tailored group', calling the efficacy of tailored communications into question. We must emphasize here that we believe that tailored communications can engender meaningful dietary change, but are not convinced that a number of alternative explanations of such effects (e.g. amount and perceived quality of information) have yet been ruled out.

These potential ambiguities are not restricted to tailored studies. For example, Schuler *et al.* (1992) recruited angina patients and randomly assigned them to an intervention or control group. Whereas the control group received their normal medical care, the intervention group stayed on a 'metabolic' ward for the first three weeks of the programme, and were given low-fat, low-cholesterol diets, group training sessions (two hours per week) and home exercise sessions (20 minutes per day). Those in the intervention group reduced their fat intake by 53 per cent, and their cholesterol by 10 per cent). Comparably, Howard-Pitney *et al.* (1997) recruited participants from low socioeconomic status groups and compared six 90-minute classes with a control group of people who received the normal nutrition curriculum. Findings indicated that those in the intervention group showed a 2.3 per cent greater reduction in the proportion of calories they derived from fat than the control condition. To put the latter figure in some perspective, if this were translated to the US population as a whole it might save up to 23,000 lives per year (Rose 1985).

Thus, there have been several attempts to change dietary behaviour, with greater effects on people the further 'downstream' the intervention. However, it is worth noting that the further downstream the intervention, the more intensive it is, making it difficult to identify the precise nature of the effects. While it is likely that the positive effects of Schuler *et al.* and Howard-Pitney *et al.* are due to the intervention, exactly what part of the intervention is having an effect? Compared with the no-treatment controls, intervention group participants are receiving more attention from health professionals, being involved in group sessions, receiving more feedback, receiving more information and having regular appointments, all of which (and more) may be beneficial to health. Moreover, from a public health perspective, these interventions can be costly and time-consuming.

In an attempt to control for the effects of presenting people with large amounts of information or high levels of personal attention, some authors have developed **minimal interventions** to investigate more closely the effects of tailoring. For example, van Buerden *et al.* (1990) compared blood cholesterol levels between people who attended cholesterol screening sites in various public venues (e.g. shopping centres) and the blood bank. Those who attended the cholesterol screening sites were given personal feedback about the level of cholesterol in their blood, as well as five suggestions for reducing fat intake; those who attended the blood bank were not even told that their cholesterol levels would be tested. Cholesterol levels were reassessed three months later. There were significant differences between the groups: cholesterol levels fell in the feedback group, but actually rose in the control group. Thus, minimal interventions can be effective in reducing cholesterol. However, as van Buerden *et al.* (1990) point out, there were some potentially serious problems with the sample. Two in particular are of note here. First, the public screening sample were self-selecting; in other words, because they volunteered to take part they might have been more motivated to change their behaviour to begin with. Second, the control sample consisted of blood donors. Given that only 55 per cent of women and 67 per cent of men are eligible to donate blood (of whom only about 8 per cent actually do so; Linden *et al.* 1988), members of this group might share certain characteristics that make them an unsuitable comparison group (e.g. they might be more 'health motivated').

More recently, Armitage and Conner (2001a) sought to address some of these difficulties by providing a minimal intervention in a more general population. The sample received the same basic nutrition information, along with a letter welcoming them to the study and thanking them for their support. The only difference between the control and experimental conditions was that the letters sent to those in the experimental condition consisted of one additional sentence, informing them of the proportion of food energies they currently derived from fat. Contrasting those currently eating a low-fat diet with those not currently eating a low-fat diet, Armitage and Conner (2001a) showed that the minimal intervention successfully reduced saturated fat intake. Framed in terms of the HBM, theory of planned behaviour and PMT, the information may have increased perceived susceptibility; framed in terms of the TTM, it might have prompted precontemplators to consider changing their diets. Thus, it seems as if tailored messages – even very brief ones – can provide important benefits and further research is required to evaluate and enhance current health promotion campaigns.

Promoting dietary change

The previous section reviewed several models of health behaviours and examined how they have contributed to our understanding of dietary change. We then examined the effects of a number of interventions, which had used variables from these models to tailor or target those interventions. It is clear that social psychology has advanced our understanding of dietary change by identifying a number of key predictors of dietary change. However, as yet, we have not considered the mechanisms by which these variables may be changed; although successful, a number of dietary interventions have been unable to identify mechanisms for change. For example, it seems likely that changing someone's attitude may help them change their diet, but how exactly would you go about changing attitude? The following section examines some of the theories underpinning general attempts to change people's cognitions and behaviours.

Personal risk information and fear appeals

From the research into tailored interventions, it seems as if providing people with personal risk information might be an effective means of changing their behaviour. Indeed, this type of approach seems to be consistent with the accounts provided by both the HBM and PMT: that perceived threat (i.e. susceptibility and severity) is a determinant of behaviour. But what is it about perceived threat that might engender change? There are two possible explanations: that personal risk information induces fear or that it challenges optimistic biases.

It seems likely that increasing people's perceptions of severity of illness and their personal susceptibility to that illness would be an effective means of changing their behaviour. For example, as we have already shown, people who eat an unhealthy diet are more susceptible to conditions such as CHD and cancer, both of which are severe. The implication is that providing people with negative personal feedback – or inducing fear in them – might be sufficient to encourage them to change. In a quantitative review of 35 studies, Sutton (1982) found a linear relationship between fear and behaviour change, such that greater fear produced more behaviour change. However, consistent with our reviews of HBM and PMT, perceived threat is often not strongly related to behaviour. Moreover, social psychologists have known for some time that the relationship between fear and propensity to act is somewhat complex and depends not just on the 'amount' of fear contained in a message, but on how the recipient reacts. For example, Janis and Feshbach (1953) systematically studied the effects of fear on the impact of health promotion messages. They found that those in the most fearful group remembered less of the information that was provided to them and that their behaviour was no different from that of the comparison groups. In fact, Janis and Feshbach (1953) were able to show that while medium levels of fear could motivate behaviour, low and high levels of fear actually demotivated people.

Under what circumstances might a fear appeal produce behaviour change? A meta-analysis of more than 100 studies investigating fear appeals sought to address this question. Witte and Allen (2000) concluded that the stronger the fear aroused by a fear appeal, the more persuasive it is, but that fear is particularly effective if it is accompanied by a message designed to induce self-efficacy. In other words, people generally react to fear appeals if they believe that they can do something to protect themselves from the threat (Sutton 1982). Similarly, personal feedback is likely to work best when accompanied with information about how to deal with the threat (e.g. Brug *et al.* 1999; Armitage and Conner 2001a). The implication is that the effectiveness of a health intervention depends upon both the message itself and the way in which it is received by the recipient (cf. PMT).

A second possible mechanism for explaining the effects of personalized feedback concerns **unrealistic optimism**. Unrealistic optimism is a bias in risk perception whereby people underestimate the chances of something negative happening to them and overestimate the extent to which positive things will happen to them (Weinstein 1980). In relation to dietary change, these people are much less likely to believe they are at risk from cardiovascular disease or cancer than are other people and are therefore much less likely to be motivated to do anything about it. Potentially, providing people with personalized feedback might counter their tendency to be optimistically biased and thereby encourage them to change their behaviour. Further research is required to target more precisely the kinds of variables that are likely to undermine optimistic bias, such as lowering people's perceived control over the health risk (e.g. Weinstein 1980; Helweg-Larsen and Shepperd 2001).

Changing attitudes

The TPB provides a useful description of the kind of information that one might include within a persuasive communication: according to Ajzen and Fishbein (1980), one changes the underlying salient beliefs in order to promote behaviour change. However, what this account does not tell us is *how* we are supposed to do this and what exactly we are trying to make people do. In other words, what goes on in people's heads when they receive this message? There are a number of models of attitude change that do precisely this, and we focus on Petty and Cacioppo's (1986) **elaboration likelihood model** (but see Chaiken 1980 for a discussion of the related heuristic-systematic model).

Petty and Cacioppo's (1986) elaboration likelihood model (ELM) is partly based on Greenwald's (1968) cognitive response model. Basically, the cognitive response model states that the more people think about a persuasive communication, the more likely they are to be persuaded by it. In other words, the more issue-relevant thoughts that a message elicits, the more likely people are to change their opinions. Petty and Cacioppo regard these **cognitive responses** as an **elaboration** of the relevant arguments and, provided that people are sufficiently motivated and generate thoughts that are consistent with the direction of the message, they will be persuaded. Thus, people are more likely to be persuaded by strong arguments than by weak arguments. Within the ELM, however, this is only one route to **persuasion**, and is known as the **central route**.

One obvious flaw in the central route to persuasion is that we are not always motivated to process messages in this depth. In fact, most of us can probably think of times when we have been persuaded to buy products on the basis of information given by someone who seems to know what they are talking about. The ELM acknowledges that people are not always motivated to process messages in a rigorous way, and propose a second, **peripheral route** to persuasion. When people are not motivated or are unable fully to process a persuasive message, Petty and Cacioppo (1986) argue that factors that have nothing to do with the presented arguments become persuasive. Among the peripheral cues that have been shown to be persuasive are the status of the communicator (attractive or expert people are generally most persuasive) and the length of the argument (long messages are more persuasive).

The ELM may therefore explain some of the effects of the large-scale interventions we described above. For instance, peripheral route processing might explain why mass media campaigns such as the one described by Reger *et al.* (1999) are sometimes effective in changing people's behaviour, even if they do not explicitly refer to social psychological theories. In addition, perhaps tailored messages (Brug *et al.* 1999), courses of action endorsed by a physician (Beresford *et al.* 1997) and personalized feedback might enhance central route processing by increasing the personal relevance of the information. Similarly, although the ELM has only really been applied to evaluate attitude change, we see no reason why the same principles could not be used to change (for example) self-efficacy or any other social cognitive variable. Further research is required to investigate these possibilities in the field of dietary change. Moreover, empirical tests of the ELM have typically been restricted to American undergraduate populations and there is only limited evidence of its generalizability at present. One really important message for the field of dietary change is that many of the dietary change attempts we have described have (at least implicitly) assumed that participants are motivated to read the information they are given and will thereby act upon it. Accumulated research into the ELM suggests this is not the case and researchers should be cognizant of this fact.

Enhancing self-efficacy

In addition to the techniques designed to change people's attitudes, Bandura (1986) provides a description of the way in which self-efficacy can be enhanced. In addition to the standard persuasive techniques discussed in relation to the ELM, Bandura (1986) elucidates three processes. The first is personal mastery, which involves the accomplishment of sub-goals; in other words, rather than trying to eat a low-fat diet immediately, one might try to choose lower-fat alternatives when given a choice. The second is modelling, or observing other people and learning about their success. The third is learning to use relaxation techniques in order to control feelings of arousal or anxiety. Interestingly, Bandura's (1986) suggestions for promoting self-efficacy could be interpreted as a distillation of Prochaska and DiClemente's (1983) ten processes of change, which similarly mix coping with temptation, goal-setting and social support. Some of the tailored interventions reviewed above (e.g. Steptoe *et al.* 1999) seem to draw on goal-setting to promote change. Similarly, Howard-Pitney *et al.* (1997) gave mastery skills, modelling and persuasive messages to their intervention group and were successful in promoting dietary change. Consistently, though, research attention has been focused on initiating behaviour, rather than on maintaining it or preventing relapse, and we have found no evidence of attempts to employ relaxation techniques to maintain behaviour.

This section has examined some of the theories that might explain the mechanisms by which successful dietary change programmes exert their effects. These mechanisms are important because, once identified, they can be targeted explicitly in the future. To date, they have been investigated on only an implicit level and further research is required to put the mechanisms into practice.

Summary and conclusions

In this chapter we have examined the powerful influence that dietary intake exerts over health, notably cardiovascular diseases and cancer, and that while people are aware of the issues, they are not generally meeting government targets. We have also reviewed a number of social psychological models that have been applied to the study of dietary change. In our view, there have been too few studies that have used such models: (a) to predict dietary change by evaluating the effectiveness of dietary interventions using social psychological models of health behaviour; or (b) to explain dietary change by targeting key variables and observing changes in subsequent behaviour. For example, in an extensive review of dietary change attempts, Kumanyika *et al.* (2000) make only passing reference to the models of health behaviour reviewed above, reflecting the dearth of social psychological research in this area. Similarly, they note that the vast majority of medical research has focused on highly motivated (usually high-risk) people and thus has very little to say about the population as a whole.

Perhaps more importantly, as we noted at the beginning of the chapter, significant health benefits are only likely to accrue over relatively long periods of time. Temple (1996) argues that consistently eating a low-fat diet over a period of five years is the only way in which one is likely to reduce one's risk of CHD. The same is true of fruit and vegetable consumption. One thing that the social psychology of dietary change currently has very little to say about is the maintenance of dietary change. In this context, the majority of studies reported in this chapter are short term and are thus unable to account for long-term change. Even the TTM, which explicitly includes a maintenance stage, conceptualizes this in terms of months (six), rather than the years that are required to confer the significant health benefits associated with dietary change. Encouragingly, new research seems to suggest that the predictive power of some key cognitions can be long term. In a recent study, Conner *et al.* (2002) examined the ability of TPB variables to predict fat and fruit and vegetable intake across a six-year period. Findings indicated that intentions were still predictive of behaviour six years later. Perhaps more importantly, Conner *et al.* (2002) showed that intention stability was an important factor: if it were possible to identify the antecedents of intention stability, it might be possible to address issues associated with the maintenance of dietary change. What is clear is that further longitudinal work into the maintenance of dietary change is required.

Rothman (2000) has also suggested the need for a social psychology of maintenance, arguing that the majority of models of health behaviour are geared towards initiating behaviour, to the detriment of maintenance. More specifically, Rothman (2000) argues that there are different processes underpinning the initiation and maintenance of a behaviour. On the one hand, the decision to initiate a behaviour is based on holding favourable expectancies regarding future outcomes; in contrast, maintaining a behaviour is more concerned with whether the outcomes associated with one's current behaviour are sufficiently satisfying to pursue the behaviour further. Moreover, Rothman (2000) suggests that this level of satisfaction depends upon comparing one's current pattern of behaviour with the potential satisfaction that might be derived from another (e.g. unhealthy) pattern of behaviour. The implication is that the long-term positive outcomes associated with (for example) eating a healthy diet are likely to be less salient than the short-term positive benefits to be derived from eating a tasty pie. This means that it is likely to prove difficult to promote long-term dietary change, although people will willingly cycle through trying (and failing) to eat a healthy diet (see Chapter 4). One possibility worth exploring is that providing people with the skills required to implement Prochaska and DiClemente's processes of change or Bandura's strategies for enhancing self-efficacy might prove effective.

We began the chapter by asking whether health was really a major determinant of dietary change. Although there is some evidence that health does motivate dietary change, it is clear that health is not the major motivator for change, at least in the short term. After all, if health were the major motivator, one might expect personal feedback to exert much greater effects on behaviour. As yet, our knowledge of the long-term consequences of dietary interventions is patchy and more research attention that tackles the problem of maintenance is required. Nevertheless, the work we have considered in this chapter shows that there are statistically and clinically significant benefits to be derived from adopting a social psychological approach to dietary change. Chapter 4 continues this theme by examining the use of social psychology to affect a very specific problem associated with dietary intake: weight loss.

Notes

1 For foodstuffs that cannot obviously be divided as such (e.g. one potato, one banana), a 'serving' or 'portion' is defined (approximately) as 120 ml (half a cup) for fruits, vegetables or pulses.
2 Armitage *et al.* (2002) argue that decisional balance and self-efficacy are equivalent to the concepts of attitude and perceived behavioural control, respectively (cf. Ajzen 1998; Duran and Trafimow 2000).

Suggested further reading

Conner, M. and Norman, P. (1996) *Predicting Health Behaviour*. Buckingham: Open University Press.
   Each chapter of this popular text reviews, critiques and tests a different social psychological model of health behaviour, many of which have examined dietary behaviours in one form or another.
Norman, P., Abraham, C. and Conner, M. (2000) *Understanding and Changing Health Behaviour: From Health Beliefs to Self-regulation*. Reading: Harwood Academic Press.
   A recent book which looks at the social psychological approach to changing health behaviour in general.
Rutter, D.R. and Quine, L. (eds) (2002) *Changing Health Behaviour: Intervention and Research with Social Cognition Models*. Buckingham: Open University Press.
   This book looks at the various social psychological approach to changing health behaviour.
Tones, K. and Tilford, S. (2001) *Health Promotion: Effectiveness, Efficiency and Equity*. Cheltenham: Nelson Thornes.
   Third edition of a well respected book that addresses issues raised in Chapter 3 from the perspective of health promotion practitioners.

4

Weight control and disorders of eating

General overview

This chapter examines the important issues of weight control, disorders of eating and the contributions that social psychology has made to furthering our understanding of these issues. A common theme running through the chapter is a focus on the amount individuals eat, the factors influencing this and the implications for their health and body weight. Hence, the key distinction from Chapter 3 is a focus on changing the amount of calories consumed rather than changing the type of foods consumed. We first examine the importance of **weight control** and its implications for health. We then examine **obesity** as an extreme example of problems with weight control. The following sections examine different strategies used to control weight and then social psychological perspectives on understanding such strategies. Finally, we examine the eating disorders of anorexia and bulimia nervosa. Understanding of the importance of the social acceptability of particular weights and body shapes has been a key contribution of social psychological approaches in this area and this work is reviewed at various points in this chapter.

The importance of weight control

At one level of analysis, weight control is simply the outcome of the balance between energy consumed and expended. If more energy is consumed than expended (a positive energy balance) the result will be weight gain; while if more energy is expended than consumed (a negative energy balance) the result will be weight loss. At a physiological level the human body is sophisticated in ensuring a balance between energy consumed and expended (i.e. maintaining energy homeostasis) through hormonal and neural signals which influence the size of meals (Garrow 1977; Woods *et al.* 2000; see Chapter 2 on the satiety cascade). However, a variety of environmental conditions can override these physiological mechanisms and lead to either a positive or negative energy balance. Where access to palatable food is readily available, as is the case in most Western societies, a negative energy balance is relatively rare and appears to be generally difficult to maintain. Anorexia nervosa is a condition characterized by a negative energy balance and low body weight. This is a potentially life threatening condition, but is fortunately uncommon. In contrast, a positive energy balance and associated excessive body weight is more common. As we shall see, a variety of factors contribute to this situation, including the high palatability of many foods.

There are a variety of definitions of body weight in relation to health outcomes. A common measure is body mass index (BMI). BMI is defined as the individual's weight (in kilograms) divided by the square of their height (in metres). Normal weights are in the range of BMIs from 18.5 to 25. Overweight is defined as a BMI between 25 and 30, while obesity is defined as a BMI of greater than 30, with moderate obesity defined as a BMI between 30 and 35, severe obesity defined as a BMI of between 35 and 40 and very severe obesity defined as a BMI in excess of 40. Similarly, underweight is defined as a BMI of less than 18.5 (International Obesity Task Force 2001). The problem with this measure is that it fails to distinguish lean body mass from stored fat and it is the stored fat levels that seem to be important in relation to health outcomes. For example, many top class rugby players have BMIs of greater than 30 despite having low levels of stored body fat. Another measure of degree of overweight or underweight compares heights and weights to those given in standard tables. These tables have been produced by life insurance companies based on information about mortality rates for men and women of different weights and heights. Typically such tables report 'healthy' weight ranges for individuals of different heights, genders and frame sizes. So, for example, the 1983 Metropolitan Life Insurance Company tables quote a healthy weight range of 155–169 pounds (70.3–76.7 kg) for a six-foot man of medium build and 130–144 pounds (59.0–65.3 kg) for a five-foot six-inch woman of medium build (Table 4.1). Overweight and underweight are then defined in relation to these healthy weight ranges. For example, one definition of obesity is where body weight is in excess of the healthy weight range by 20 per cent or more. Other measures use more direct estimates of the percentage of body fat. Table 4.2 shows the estimated percentage body fat for African Americans and whites of different ages, genders and BMIs (Gallagher *et al.* 2000). For example, the average 50-year-old male with a BMI in excess of 30 is predicted to have 28 per cent body fat.

Examination of the distribution of body weight across the population in relation to these ideals is quite illuminating. It has been estimated that about 20 per cent of the US population between the ages of 30 and 62 years have a BMI of 30 or more (Jeffery *et al.* 2000). A total of 24 per cent of men and 27 per cent of women in the USA are obese (≥20 per cent above desirable weight; Kuczmarski *et al.* 1994) and the prevalence has doubled since 1900.

Table 4.1 Metropolitan Life Insurance Company recommended weights for different heights and frame sizes for men and women aged 25–59

| Height | *Healthy weight range in pounds* | | | | | |
| | *Small frame* | | *Medium frame* | | *Large frame* | |
(feet and inches)	*Men*	*Women*	*Men*	*Women*	*Men*	*Women*
4 9		99–108		106–118		115–128
4 10		100–110		108–120		117–131
4 11		101–112		110–123		119–134
5 0		103–115		112–126		122–137
5 1	123–129	105–118	126–136	115–129	133–145	125–140
5 2	125–131	108–121	128–138	118–132	122–137	128–144
5 3	127–133	111–124	130–140	121–135	125–141	131–148
5 4	129–135	114–127	132–143	124–138	128–145	134–152
5 5	131–137	117–130	134–146	127–141	131–149	137–156
5 6	133–140	120–133	137–149	130–144	135–154	140–160
5 7	135–143	123–136	140–152	133–147	140–159	143–164
5 8	137–146	126–139	143–155	136–150	144–163	146–167
5 9	139–149	129–142	146–158	139–153	148–167	149–170
5 10	141–152	132–145	149–161	142–156	152–172	152–173
5 11	144–155		152–165		157–177	
6 0	147–159		155–169		161–182	
6 1	150–163		159–173		166–187	
6 2	153–167		162–177		171–192	
6 3	157–171		166–182		175–197	

Source: Metropolitan Life Insurance Company 1983. Reproduced with permission

Table 4.2 Predicted percentage body fat by sex for African-Americans and whites

| | *Age (years)* | | |
	20–39	*40–59*	*60–79*
Men			
BMI < 18.5	8	11	13
BMI ≥ 25	20	22	25
BMI ≥ 30	25	28	30
Women			
BMI < 18.5	21	23	24
BMI ≥ 25	33	34	36
BMI ≥ 30	39	40	42

Source: Gallagher *et al.* 2000. Reproduced with permission

In the UK, obesity levels have also increased in recent years. In 1980, 6 per cent of men and 8 per cent of women had BMIs in excess of 30. By 1995, 15 per cent of men and 17 per cent of women were estimated to have BMIs in excess of 30 (White *et al.* 1991; International Obesity Task Force 2001). Obesity levels are particularly high in minority and low socioeconomic status groups (Sobal and Stunkard 1989) and prevalence increases with age, particularly among women. Together these risk factors can lead to very high rates of obesity. For example, 60 per cent of African-American women between the ages of 45 and 75 years are obese (van Itallie 1985), while 77 per cent of Western Samoan women between the ages of 25 and 69 were reported to be obese in 1991 (International Obesity Task Force 2001). The increasing rates of obesity are probably partly attributable to *both* reductions in energy expenditure through physical activity and an increasing consumption of calories as appetizing but energy-dense foods. The high palatability of many foods and their high fat content (fat contains more energy than the same weight of carbohydrate or protein) are both associated with additional consumption. Overweight and obesity are associated with a range of health problems, including hypertension, diabetes, cancer and heart disease. However, there is considerable debate about the precise relationship between degree of overweight and risk. Risks of various health problems are estimated to be elevated at weights that are anything from 5 to 25 per cent above ideal and to rise gradually with increasing degree of overweight above these levels (Brownell and Rodin 1994). Given the severity of the health problems associated with greater levels of excess weight and the large percentage of individuals classified as obese, the factors influencing weight control have been a major focus of research attention.

Another major factor influencing interest in weight control and eating disorders has been the importance currently placed upon a slim body shape in many cultures. In Western cultures, in particular, a limited range of body shapes are deemed acceptable, particularly for women (Rothblum 1990; Grogan 1999). Being overweight is viewed negatively, even by overweight individuals (Tiggemann 1992). For women slimness is particularly valued, while for men a mesomorphic and muscular shape is considered most acceptable (Lamb *et al.* 1993). This has been true since at least the 1960s, although the ideal for women has become consistently leaner and is now much thinner than what is most appropriate in terms of health outcomes (Brownell and Wadden 1992). The changes in what body shape is considered most acceptable support the idea that such ideals are driven more by cultural ideals than what is to be preferred on health grounds.

A considerable body of social psychological research has demonstrated prejudice against individuals who do not conform to these ideal body shapes (Crandall 1994). Cash (1990) reviews evidence showing that this prejudice begins in childhood, with children preferring not to play with overweight peers and assigning negative adjectives to drawings of overweight individuals. In adulthood, overweight individuals tend to be rated as less active and athletic, but also less intelligent, hardworking, successful and popular (see Chapter 6). They also experience prejudice in relation to getting places in good colleges and getting good jobs. Tiggemann and Rothblum (1988) showed that American and Australian college students shared similar negative stereotypes of overweight individuals, particularly women. Such negative views of the overweight appear to be particularly common in individualistic cultures where individuals are held to be responsible for their own fates (i.e. for being overweight; Crandall and Martinez 1996).

One impact of the current acceptability of a slim body shape is the popularity of dieting and other weight control strategies as one way to attain that shape. Much previous research in this area has assumed that dieting is principally based upon dissatisfaction with current body weight and shape (Grogan 1999). This dissatisfaction is assumed to originate from the mismatch between individuals' current body weight and shape and the slim ideals prominent in our culture. Dieting is seen as the best way to achieve the culturally valued outcome of an acceptably slim body shape. One possible mechanism by which the media might influence body dissatisfaction is via acting as a source of slim ideals against which unfavourable self-comparisons are made (Richins 1991; Grogan et al. 1996). This process is referred to as upward social comparison, because one's own body shape is compared unfavourably with slim ideals presented in the media. Social psychologists have also been prominent in examining the role of the media in promoting different body images (Grogan 1999). For example, Silverstein et al. (1986) noted that the media reflect the fact that the pressure on women to have a slim body shape is greater than that on men. They reported that a content analysis of 33 television shows revealed 69 per cent of female characters to be thin and only 5 per cent to be heavy. In contrast, only 18 per cent of men were thin, while 26 per cent were heavy. Similar patterns are evident in magazines, particularly those aimed at women. Grogan et al. (1996) directly examined the impact of viewing same-gender, slim, conventionally attractive media images on the body satisfaction of women and men. Compared to a control group, both women's and men's satisfaction with their own body shape decreased significantly immediately after viewing the media images. This research would suggest that body dissatisfaction may be particularly common among those likely to engage in such upward social comparison. Various studies in Western societies demonstrate high levels of dissatisfaction with body shape, particularly among women, and that dissatisfaction may begin from as early as ten years of age (Pliner et al. 1990; Tiggemann and Pennington 1990; Conner et al. 1996). Such dissatisfaction may lead to subsequent attempts to change one's body shape so that it matches the idealized images presented in the media, and so to reduce body dissatisfaction (Garner et al. 1980; Itzin 1986). However, for most individuals such body shapes are unattainable, leading to further dissatisfaction with their body shape. This dissatisfaction may have an important role to play in the development of eating disorders.

Obesity

Obesity is defined as an unhealthy amount of body fat (Jeffery *et al.* 2000). The exact amount of fat defined as unhealthy has been a matter of some debate. Nevertheless, obesity is associated with higher rates of mortality and morbidity. The greater the obesity, the greater the risk. The increased mortality is largely accounted for by early death from coronary heart disease, diabetes mellitus, digestive diseases and cancers (Gilbert 1989). Fat carried in the upper body, particularly around the stomach, appears to be associated with greater risk than fat carried in the lower body (Brownell and Wadden 1992). Human obesity represents a complex disorder of multiple origin, including genetic disposition, diverse health behaviours and individual food choices (Drewnowski 1996). Indeed, there may be various different forms of obesity, each with different causes (Brownell and Wadden 1992). The development of obesity is influenced by familial risk and can be moderated by changes in energy intake, physical activity and energy expenditure. However, despite intensive research effort it is clear that we still do not have a good understanding of the precise relationship between these variables and the development of obesity. In this section, we review some of the evidence about genetic disposition and various eating behaviours as determinants of obesity. The section ends with a brief review of treatments for obesity, an issue that is given more detailed consideration in the next section on more general weight control strategies.

Although it is clear that the causes of obesity are wide-ranging, there is clearly a genetic element to obesity. For example, approximately 40 per cent of children with one obese parent become obese, while approximately 70 per cent of children with two obese parents become obese themselves. Nevertheless, it is not clear how much this is attributable to genetic factors and how much to children learning inappropriate eating and exercise patterns from their parents. In addition, Stunkard *et al.* (1990) reported that genetic factors accounted for 66–70 per cent of the variance in body mass index in 93 identical twins reared apart and presumably exposed to different eating and exercise patterns. It is thought that genetic factors may exert their influence by determining the number and distribution of adipose cells which store fat in the body. These fat cells are thought to be related to the body weight set point (Nisbett 1972). The body weight set point is the weight the body's physiological mechanisms attempt to maintain against increase or decrease. This is probably linked to the amount of fat stored in the body. When the fat cells are 'full', hunger is reduced. Thus being born with fewer adipose cells may mean that hunger is reduced when the amount of stored body fat is at a lower level (i.e. a lower set point). Although the numbers of adipose cells cannot decrease, they can increase with weight gain (Bjorntorp 1987). This may lead to an increased set point, making future weight loss more difficult to sustain. Nevertheless, several researchers make it clear that genetic factors lead only to a vulnerability to develop obesity. Lower calorie intake and regular physical activity can still prevent its onset (Brownell and Wadden 1992). For example, the similarity in weight (the concordance) is substantially higher in lighter (60 per cent) than in heavier (36 per cent) twins (Price and Stunkard 1989).

Another important factor in obesity is energy expenditure. Energy expenditure appears to be principally the result of three processes: basal metabolic rate, energy used in physical activity and thermogenesis (the production of body heat). If any of these processes uses less energy a positive energy balance may be created despite lack of change in eating patterns, and weight gain will be the result. Resting metabolic rate accounts for 60–75 per cent of daily energy expenditure in sedentary individuals (Brownell and Wadden 1992). Lower metabolic rates are indeed associated with a tendency to become obese (Ravussin et al. 1988). Metabolic rate is influenced by a range of factors, including genetics. Some individuals may inherit a tendency to have a slower metabolic rate, which may make them prone to weight gain. Metabolic rate can also be influenced by reduced food intake or dieting and by exercise. For example, dieting behaviours (i.e. restraint) can result in long-term reductions in metabolic rate. Exercise may be a particularly important method of weight control because energy is directly used in the exercise and additional energy is used through the increase in metabolic rate following exercise. We consider exercise and other methods of controlling or decreasing body weight in a later section.

Thermogenesis was the third method of energy expenditure just mentioned. Food consumption (particularly of high carbohydrate foods) leads to increased thermogenesis (Jequier 1987). This appears to be one way in which body weight is maintained at a constant level despite changes in food intake. One suggestion is that thermogenesis is impaired in obese individuals (Schwartz et al. 1985), perhaps because of lower levels of brown adipose tissue, which appears to have a role in this process. However, such processes have not as yet been confirmed.

A common view of obesity would suggest that the eating behaviour of obese and non-obese individuals differs in various ways. In particular, that obesity results from overeating. However, Spitzer and Rodin (1981) have noted the lack of evidence for clear differences in the eating behaviours of lean and obese individuals. This finding appeared to be true of both observational and self-report studies (see Brownell and Wadden 1992). This has led to suggestions that the excess body fat that distinguishes the obese is the result of more efficient energy use in these individuals. However, more sophisticated measurement techniques (e.g. the use of more accurate 24-hour energy expenditure measures based on doubly labelled water) have indicated that in fact the obese expend more energy than do the non-obese. In addition, these techniques reveal that the obese and non-obese underestimate their daily caloric intake, but that this bias is greater in the obese (Brownell and Wadden 1992). Thus, while it is evidently true that obese individuals must at some point have maintained a positive energy balance in order to become obese (i.e. in the so-called dynamic phase of obesity), there is little evidence of significant differences in eating behaviours of obese and lean groups. It would appear likely that individuals in the static phase of obesity (where weight is not changing) are not eating differently from their lean counterparts in terms of energy balance.

There is also relatively little evidence that obese individuals have clearly distinguishable eating styles (Stunkard 1982). An early attempt to understand the basis of obesity suggested that overweight individuals were more likely to respond to stressful or emotional stimuli by eating because they had not learned to distinguish between hunger and anxiety (Kaplan and Kaplan 1957). This research is considered in more detail in Chapter 5. Reviews of the research suggest only modest support for this so-called psychosomatic theory of obesity (Greeno and Wing 1994). More importantly, Baucom and Aiken (1981) demonstrated that it was dieting rather than obesity that was the key predictor of eating in response to stress in their study. Given the fact that many obese individuals are dieting in an attempt to control their weight, this may explain why stress leads to greater eating in the obese compared to the non-obese group. Thus restraint (i.e. dieting) was suggested as a mechanism explaining overeating and obesity.

The concept of restrained eating developed from the 'set point' theory of obesity (Nisbett 1972; Herman and Polivy 1975). This theory suggests that individuals have a set point body weight that is physiologically maintained and may be genetically determined. To get to and maintain a body weight below their set point, individuals must restrain their eating. Restrained eaters are assumed to attempt to restrict their food intake through various self-control processes. However, when these self-control processes are undermined, disinhibition of eating occurs, and excessive food intake takes place. For example, restrained eaters appear not to adjust their food intake for previous food intake (Herman and Mack 1975). Unrestrained eaters adjust for consuming a 'preload' of food by eating less in a subsequent eating test; restrained eaters do not appear to perform this adjustment and eat just as much as if they had not eaten the preload. It is believed that the preload disinhibits the restraint over eating they normally show. In relation to obesity, it is suggested that restraint may actually be a determinant of obesity. This might occur in at least two ways. First, restraint may negatively impact on metabolic rate, leading to less output of energy. Second, disinhibition of eating when attempts at self-control of food intake are overridden may lead to an increased energy intake. Together these factors can lead to a positive energy balance and weight gain (Gilbert 1989). This is consistent with a series of recent studies showing that 25–45 per cent of obese individuals treated in weight control programmes report problemmes with binge eating (i.e. the consumption of large quantities of food in a small amount of time; see Brownell and Wadden 1992), often preceded by periods of restraint. Obese binge eaters are different from individuals with bulimia nervosa (see below) because they do not engage in purging (through vomiting or use of laxatives). Recent research has also suggested that the weight variability associated with varying spells of restraint and breaking restraint is itself associated with negative health outcomes (Lissner *et al.* 1991).

Another factor considered as an influence on weight control was the type of food consumed. Schachter (1971) suggested that an important factor in obesity was degree of responsiveness to the attractiveness of the food. In his externality theory, he suggested that individuals vary along a dimension he called external eating. Those low in external eating tend to start and cease eating based on internal cues of hunger. In contrast, those high in external eating are not as responsive to these internal cues and instead rely upon external cues, such as the perceived attractiveness of the food. When faced with attractive food these individuals will be more likely to overeat and thus gain weight. Schachter (1971) reported that external eating was more common in the obese and might be a causal factor. However, Rodin (1981) reported that individuals high in externality could be found at all weight levels, but that some successfully employ strategies to avoid gaining weight. Despite the appeal of this hypothesis and some supportive data, it has become clear that degree of externality is not well correlated with body weight (Rodin 1981).

In conclusion, it would appear that various studies on eating styles have generally failed to establish consistent obese versus lean differences. This would also appear to be the case for differences between such groups in attitudes towards food and food preferences (Drewnowski 1996). Further research is required to increase our understanding of the role of various behaviours in the development and maintenance of obesity.

A range of methods for treating obesity have been proposed. These include methods specific to treating obesity, which are briefly considered here, and methods used in both obese and overweight groups to control or reduce body weight. These latter methods are considered in some detail in the next section. Perhaps the most drastic intervention to reduce weight in the obese is gastric surgery. In this procedure the stomach is surgically reduced in size (usually by stapling off part of it). This procedure is not without risks and tends only to be used where the level of obesity is life threatening. Nevertheless, the procedure can be very effective in reducing weight for some individuals. Other commonly used procedures have included wiring of the jaw to reduce food intake and pharmacological treatments. However, these procedures tend to be employed only when other weight control strategies have failed (Brownell and Wadden 1992). The next section considers these strategies.

Weight control strategies

Over the past few years increasing average body weight and preferences for slimmer body shapes have been paralleled by increasing efforts aimed at weight control (Brownell and Rodin 1994; French and Jeffery 1994). While this is partly due to health concerns, achieving a socially acceptable slim body shape is often a more important outcome for many individuals. However, the role of various behaviours in the attainment and maintenance of a desirable weight and body shape is not well understood. These efforts to control weight take a variety of forms and often meet with varying degress of success in terms of initial weight loss and the amount of time for which weight loss is maintained. The determinants of these behaviours have not been widely studied. A great many weight control strategies may be effective in producing short-term (less than six months) weight reduction. However, it is strategies that can produce long-term (greater than six months) weight reduction which are of particular interest to researchers because it is with long-term control of weight that the largest health benefits are associated. In this section we review evidence concerning the effectiveness of different strategies, focusing in particular on long-term weight loss.

The majority of weight control strategies involve attempts to change individuals' energy balance by decreasing energy intake and increasing energy expenditure. Attempts to decrease energy intake take a variety of forms, including a focus on reducing total energy intake or reducing the intake of energy from fat. Drug medication has been employed to promote such reduced food intake. Increasing energy expenditure focuses on increasing physical activity levels and exercise. However, a diverse range of other behaviours, such as increasing consumption of fruit and vegetables or avoiding between-meal snacking, are likely to be considered by those attempting to control body weight and shape (Lowe 1993).

There are a range of specific maintenance strategies which have been employed in order to help individuals to maintain a weight loss. For example, very low calorie diets have been employed to encourage increased initial weight loss, particularly in obese individuals. In such diets, individuals are required to reduce calorie intake to a very low level (i.e. between 600 and 800 kcal/day) and maintain this for prolonged periods (e.g. between two and three months). Such diets have been demonstrated to produce larger weight losses than normal reduced calorie diets (i.e. usually between 1000 and 1200 kcal/day), but have little effect on long-term maintenance of weight loss (Jeffery *et al.* 2000). A more widely used strategy is the use of low-fat diets. Such diets can in themselves be beneficial for health (see Chapter 3). However, low-fat diets may also promote weight loss because fat requires less energy to metabolize and reductions in the energy derived from fat do not appear to be wholly compensated for (Brownell and Wadden 1992). However, there is little evidence that weight loss strategies focusing on reducing fat intake are considerably more successful than strategies focusing on reducing overall calorie intake. Another strategy that has been employed with more success involves increasing the length of whatever treatment is employed. Perri *et al.* (1989) demonstrated that a 40-week treatment programme was more effective in both producing and maintaining weight loss than a 20-week programme.

An increased focus on physical activity, including exercise behaviours, is another useful strategy to promote weight loss. It would appear that the greatest health benefits are associated with a change from low to moderate levels of physical activity rather than with becoming extremely active (Wood *et al.* 1991). Increased physical activity is associated with both greater initial weight loss and a slowing of weight regain (Jeffery *et al.* 2000). However, the factors promoting long-term maintenance of increased physical activity are not, as yet, well understood (Marcus *et al.* 2000). A further useful method is the use of coping skills and problem-solving strategies when problems with weight loss are encountered. The relapse prevention model of Marlatt and Gordon (1985) has stimulated interventions of this type. The individual is taught to identify situations in which lapses in behavioural adherence (to weight control behaviours) are likely to occur. Strategies to avoid such lapses or to get back on track after such a lapse has occurred are also taught. For example, in those groups who have a tendency to engage in binge eating, strategies to help individuals to resist binges can be useful for both preventing binges and promoting weight loss (Brownell and Wadden 1992). However, few studies have explicitly tested the efficacy of such approaches independently of other forms of intervention (Jeffery *et al.* 2000).

Booth and colleagues (Blair *et al.* 1989, 1990; Booth *et al.* 1989) have examined a broader range of weight control behaviours used by women attempting to lose weight. They found that attaining and maintaining an acceptable body weight was associated with the adoption of particular behavioural strategies and the avoidance of others. Taking exercise, avoiding calories between meals and avoiding emotional eating were each related to weight loss, but only avoiding calories between meals was related to maintaining a weight loss. Conner and Norman (1996) examined a similar set of weight control behaviours (limiting food intake at meals, avoiding dietary fat, taking exercise, avoiding alcohol and avoiding snacks between meals) in a sample of men and women. Each of the five behaviours was viewed as being effective in controlling body weight and shape and was performed more frequently when trying to control weight or shape than when not so trying (especially for dieters), the differences being particularly large for limiting intake at meals. However, only limiting intake and avoiding alcohol were significantly related to current body weight. Those limiting intake when trying to control weight actually tended to be heavier, have a higher maximum BMI and be more in excess of their ideal weight. In contrast, avoiding alcohol appeared to be associated with a lower current body weight. Hence, the data of Conner and Norman (1996) suggest that the restriction of intake at meals is negatively related to long-term successful weight control and shows no relationship with short-term weight loss. Such findings parallel the moderate positive correlation reported between dietary restraint measures and current BMI (e.g. Hill *et al.* 1991), which presumably better reflects the success of long-term rather than short-term weight control. In the Conner and Norman (1996) study, only avoiding alcohol showed a significant negative relationship with current weight. One explanation of this finding is provided by the results of de Castro *et al.* (1990). In studying the meal sizes of 78 normal weight adults over a one-week period, they found that meals accompanied by alcohol were significantly larger (more calories from each macronutrient) than meals eaten without alcohol. Thus, in addition to contributing calories to the diet, alcohol, at least when consumed with meals, may increase the consumption of calories from other sources, and these additional calories may contribute to problems of weight control. These findings point to the desirability of examining a broader range of weight control behaviours than is common in many studies, to further our understanding of body weight and shape control in the general population. Future research might usefully address how such behaviours relate to attaining and maintaining desirable weight (i.e. a weight/ shape the individual feels happy with and/or a weight within a healthy range), rather than simple BMI.

In summary, it would appear that we do not as yet have a good understanding of the best strategy to adopt in order to promote long-term weight loss (Jeffery *et al.* 2000). Part of the problem appears to be that we do not fully understand the factors that promote maintenance of the behaviours required for good weight control over prolonged periods of time. However, this is an area where social psychology is beginning to make a useful contribution, as the next section illustrates.

Social psychology and weight control

Social psychological research has contributed to our understanding of weight control behaviours in relation to developing theoretical models of the factors important to behaviour change and the long-term maintenance of behaviours underlying weight loss (Brownell and Wadden 1992). For example, there is evidence that increased motivation and social support can contribute to weight loss maintenance (Jeffery *et al.* 2000). In relation to attempts to control weight, the theory of reasoned action (TRA; Fishbein and Ajzen 1975) and the theory of planned behaviour (TPB; Ajzen 1991; see Chapter 2) have been applied in several studies (Schifter and Ajzen 1985; Netemeyer *et al.* 1991; Bagozzi and Kimmel 1995; Conner and Norman 1996).

The TPB is intended to provide good predictions of the decision to perform a range of behaviours, including those that are directed towards achieving goals such as weight loss. These are referred to as goal-directed behaviours (Bagozzi 1992). A goal-directed behaviour is an action a person desires to perform under the self-assumption that impediments are likely to counteract, but not necessarily thwart, any effort to act (Bagozzi and Warshaw 1990). Two classes of goal-directed behaviours are distinguished by Bagozzi. Intermediate goal-directed behaviours are problematic actions needed to achieve a desired end state (or outcome) (e.g. exercising in an attempt to lose weight). Consequence-based goal-directed behaviours are actions sought as ends in themselves (e.g.

exercise as an experiential goal, rather than as a means to another goal such as weight loss). While Ajzen argues that the TPB will be applicable to both forms of behaviours, Bagozzi (1992) and Fishbein (1993) suggest the need to examine component behaviours in attempting to predict goal achievement. Thus Ajzen would argue that we can gain an understanding of the cognitive determinants of weight control by focusing on the cognitions associated with this goal. In contrast, Bagozzi and Fishbein would suggest that we can best understand weight control by focusing on the cognitive determinants of the goal-directed behaviours employed to control weight (see Chapter 2).

Fishbein (1993) argues that it remains to be demonstrated that intention and perceived behavioural control (the proximal predictors of behaviour in the TPB) towards a goal such as weight loss are more predictive of actual weight loss than consideration of these cognitions towards each component behaviour relevant to achieving that goal. For example, an early study employing the TRA found that intentions to lose weight only correlated weakly with actual weight loss (Sejwacz *et al.* 1980). However, weight loss was somewhat better predicted by application of the TRA to the component behaviours necessary for weight loss (e.g. avoiding high-calorie foods, exercise) (Sejwacz *et al.* 1980). While three studies (Schifter and Ajzen 1985; Netemeyer *et al.* 1991; Bagozzi and Kimmel 1995) have successfully applied the TPB to predicting weight loss, none compared the application of the TPB to the outcome with its application to the component behaviours. Hence, both Bagozzi and Fishbein suggest the need to examine cognitions in relation to the component behaviours, rather than the goal itself, in attempting to predict goal achievement.

Conner and Norman (1996) examined the predictive power of the TPB in relation to the goal of weight loss and five component behaviours. It was found that intentions to limit intake, avoid fat and avoid snacks were primarily determined by attitudes, while intentions to exercise and avoid alcohol were primarily determined by perceived behavioural control. Thus attempts to change intentions to engage in these behaviours might usefully focus upon either changing attitudes or changing perceptions of control as appropriate. For the intention to pursue the goal of losing weight, consistent with the TPB, attitudes, subjective norms and perceived behavioural control were significant predictors. This goal intention was most closely related to perceived control. Thus, in terms of predicting intentions, the TPB appears equally applicable to predicting intentions to perform goal-directed behaviours or to pursue goals. The TPB data also demonstrated that performance of these five body weight and shape control behaviours was determined by both intentions and perceived control (except in the case of avoiding alcohol where attitudes displaced intentions). Thus attempts to change these behaviours would be likely to be most effective if they tackled both these components.

The data of Conner and Norman (1996) do not definitely distinguish whether application of the TPB to the goal of weight loss or to the component behaviours is the more effective means of predicting the achievement of a goal such as weight loss. However, when the amount of weight lost at last dieting episode was examined, neither intentions to lose weight nor perceived behavioural control over losing weight were significant predictors. However, intention to avoid between-meal snacks was a significant predictor, explaining 23 per cent of the variance in weight loss. This is comparable to the 19 per cent in weight loss explained by Schifter and Ajzen (1985) in their prospective study based on intentions and perceived behavioural control over weight loss. Hence, the data of Conner and Norman (1996) indicate that the prediction of the achievement of the goal of weight loss was significantly improved by application of the TPB to the component behaviours compared to its application to the goal itself. This supports the idea that goal achievement is best understood by examining component behaviours and their underlying cognitions, as Bagozzi (1992) and Fishbein (1993) suggest. Other research has similarly suggested that goal intentions (e.g. the intention to lose weight) are determined by desires, self-efficacy towards the goal, superordinate goals, relationships between superordinate goals and plans (Gollwitzer 1996; Bagozzi and Edwards 1998).

Bagozzi (1992) has also developed a theory of trying, which describes the influences upon the decision to try and actual trying to achieve a particular goal. These variables are assumed by Bagozzi to replace intention and behaviour in the TPB. Trying is held to be the more relevant variable to predict because behaviour can be successful or unsuccessful without the determining factors being any different. Moreover, particularly in relation to intermediate goal-directed behaviour, intentions can be formed towards a range of ways or means of attempting to achieve a goal and one must select among these means. This distinction is similar to Gollwitzer's (1990) distinction between goal intention (i.e. intention to try to achieve a goal) and behavioural intention (i.e. intention to achieve a goal via a specific means). Bagozzi (1992) suggests that decisions about the means to achieve a goal are determined by three interrelated processes. First, there are specific self-efficacy considerations. Means that individuals do not perceive themselves as capable of performing are less likely to be adopted, whereas means that individuals perceive to be easily executable are more likely to be performed. Self-efficacy in this scheme is very similar to perceived behavioural control in the TPB. Second, instrumental beliefs (or outcome expectancies) will play a role such that only means perceived to be likely to lead to the desired outcome or goal are likely to be adopted. Third, the desirability of or affect towards the means will play a role. More desirable means are more likely to be adopted, while noxious means are likely to be avoided. The outcome of these processes is the choice among means and subsequent attempts to perform these actions in pursuit of the goal. Presumably, successful goal achievement is dependent upon the selection of means that are indeed efficacious in achieving the goal.

Bagozzi and Edwards (2000) have tested this model in relation to the regulation of body weight. The model they tested is shown in Figure 4.1. Their model suggests that the three appraisal processes (self-efficacy, instrumental

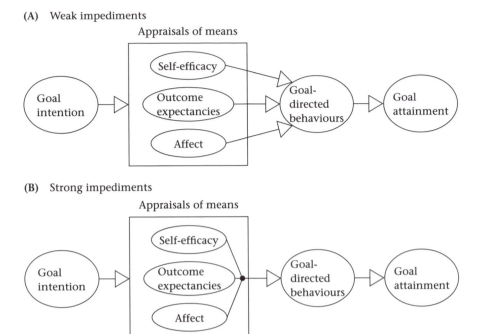

Figure 4.1 The role of appraisals on mean in the implementation of goal intentions under weak and strong impediment conditions
Source: Bagozzi and Edwards 2000. Redrawn with permission.

beliefs, affect) act either additively or interactively to determine one's choice of means to an end, depending on the perceived difficulty of initiating the behaviour. Where there are few internal or external impediments (i.e. the goal-directed behaviour is perceived as easy to perform) it is proposed that the three appraisal processes act additively. So, the more the action is seen as being within one's capabilities, as leading to the intended outcome and as being enjoyable or pleasant, the more likely is it to be engaged in. In contrast, where there are strong internal or external impediments to the action (i.e. the behaviour is seen as difficult) it is proposed that the three processes act interactively. So, the behaviour is only likely to be engaged in where all three appraisal processes are high (i.e. supportive of the behaviour). Bagozzi and Edwards (2000) tested these predictions in relation to young men and women engaging in a range of dieting or exercising behaviours designed to reduce or maintain their weight. It was predicted that dieting behaviours would generally be perceived to be easier than exercise. In addition, it was predicted that exercise behaviours would be particularly difficult for women because of the lack of support for such behaviours in the North American culture in which the model was tested.

As predicted, Bagozzi and Edwards (2000) found that for both dieting and exercising behaviours, self-efficacy, outcome expectancy or affect towards the means were sufficient to initiate action (i.e. an additive model). Self-efficacy in particular was an important determinant of all the dieting and exercising behaviours examined. The formation of intentions, strengthening of commitment and maintaining behaviour over time are all increased with high levels of self-efficacy. And this effect has been demonstrated for both dieting (Shannon *et al.* 1990) and exercise (McAuley 1993) behaviours. However, when exercise behaviours in women were examined separately by Bagozzi and Edwards, a three-way interaction was found for self-efficacy, outcome expectancy and affect. Participation by women in exercise and sporting activities as a means for body weight control occurs only when self-efficacy, outcome expectancy and affect towards means are jointly favourable.

Thus this research would point to the importance of a number of cogitive factors in weight control. A strong motivation or intention to control one's weight is important, but only in terms of providing the motivation to engage in weight control behaviours. In terms of which behaviours are engaged in to control weight, feeling confident that one can perform the behaviour (i.e. self-efficacy) is particularly important. Where the behaviour is difficult, perceiving the behaviour to lead to favoured outcomes (e.g. weight loss) and enjoying the behaviour are also important. These variables could provide important targets for interventions designed to increase weight control efforts. Nevertheless, they tell us relatively little about the factors important in maintaining these behaviours over the prolonged periods that might be necessary to maintain a healthy body weight. It may be that maintenance is simply a function of retaining a strong motivation or intention to control one's weight. For example, having stable intentions is predictive of eating a low-fat diet (Conner *et al.* 2000) or eating healthily over a prolonged period (Conner *et al.* 2002). Similarly, retaining a strong, stable feeling of self-efficacy about performing a behaviour is likely to be important (Conner *et al.* 2000). It may also be the case that certain individuals are better able to maintain a particular pattern of behaviour because of particular personality traits they possess. For example, individuals high on the personality dimension of conscientiousness are thought to be more organized, careful, dependable, self-disciplined and achievement-oriented (McCrae and John 1992). There is also evidence that they tend to adopt problem-focused rather than emotion-focused coping responses (Watson and Hubbard 1996) and that they are less likely to use escape-avoidance strategies (O'Brien and Delongis 1996). Thus conscientiousness may result in greater planfulness (Conner and Abraham 2001) and so promote both initiation and maintenance of weight control behaviours, intention formation and behaviour.

There have also been recent attempts to develop theories of the factors important to the maintenance of a behaviour. For example, the relapse prevention model of Marlatt and Gordon (1985) has stimulated theoretical developments in relation to the understanding of long-term weight control

(Brownell and Wadden 1992; Jeffery *et al.* 2000). Similarly, the transtheoretical model of change (Prochaska *et al.* 1992; see Chapter 3) highlights how different factors may be important in initially losing weight and then maintaining this weight loss. Basic to these theories is the idea that different factors may be important in the decision to initiate a behaviour and maintain a behaviour. The TPB or Bagozzi's theory of trying appear to give a good account of the variables important in the decision to initiate a behaviour like dieting. However, different factors or the same factors acting via different processes may be important in determining the decision to maintain a behaviour. For example, satisfaction with the outcome of the behaviour (e.g. weight loss) may be important in the decision to maintain, but not initiate, a behaviour (Rothman 2000). In contrast, self-efficacy may be an important determinant of both initiation and maintenance of weight control behaviours, but act in different ways (Bandura 2001). Similarly, social support appears to be an important predictor of initial weight loss attempts and longer-term maintenance (Wing *et al.* 1991). In terms of initiation, social support may need to take the form of encouragement from others to try weight loss behaviours, while in terms of maintenance, social support may need to take the form of knowing others with whom to perform the behaviour (e.g. people to go to the exercise class with).

Schwarzer's health action process approach (Schwarzer 1992; Schwarzer and Fuchs 1996) provides one account of how self-efficacy might influence maintenance of a behaviour. He suggests that successful maintenance is dependent on the implementation of an action plan that includes a set of cognitive and behavioural skills that help people cope with behavioural lapses, and thus prevent complete relapse of the behaviour. Rothman (2000) suggests that the decisions to initiate and to maintain a behaviour are based upon outcome expectancies. However, the key distinction between initiation and maintenance of a behaviour is that the former is an approach behaviour, while the latter is an avoidance behaviour. Thus the decision to initiate a behaviour is based on a consideration of the potential benefits afforded by the new pattern of behaviour compared to the current situation (i.e. outcome expectancies). Initiating a new behaviour thus depends on holding favourable expectancies regarding future outcomes. In relation to reducing one's weight the expectancies might include being able to wear new clothes, or feeling more physically confident. Because the process of behavioural initiation can be conceptualized as the attempt to reduce the discrepancy between a current state and a desired reference state, it can be viewed as an approach-based self-regulatory system (Carver and Scheier 1990). In contrast, decisions to maintain a behaviour involve decisions as to whether the outcomes associated with the new pattern of behaviour are sufficiently desirable to warrant continued action. Thus, the decision to maintain a behaviour depends principally on perceived satisfaction with received outcomes. In relation to having reduced one's weight the received outcomes might include the extent to which one feels physically confident or receives compliments on one's body shape. Because the process of behavioural maintenance can be conceptualized as the attempt to maintain the discrepancy between a current state and an undesired reference state, it can be viewed as an avoidance-based self-regulatory system (Carver and Scheier 1990).

If the decision to maintain a behaviour is principally based on satisfaction with received outcomes, we might ask what determines satisfaction. Rothman (2000) suggests that satisfaction will depend upon comparisons of received outcomes with expectations about what rewards a new pattern of behaviour will provide. So, for example, if one expectation is that one will receive many compliments for a reduced body weight obtained through dieting, the extent to which one does or does not receive these compliments will influence the decision to continue to diet or not. An important implication of this model is that interventions that heighten expectations may be useful in initiating behaviour change but be detrimental to the maintenance of a behaviour. It will be interesting to see if these predictions are borne out by future empirical studies. Indeed, more generally there is a need to demonstrate that interventions designed to target the factors identified in these theoretical models of the initiation and maintenance of behaviour do indeed produce increased initiation and maintenance of weight control behaviours.

Eating disorders

There are a number of disorders of eating. In this section we consider two such disorders: **anorexia nervosa** and **bulimia nervosa**. Anorexia nervosa and bulimia nervosa are disorders characterized by abnormal patterns of eating behaviour and body weight regulation accompanied by disturbance in perceptions of body shape and attitudes towards weight and shape (American Psychiatric Association 1994). Low self-esteem, depression and anxiety are common in both disorders. In addition, between 90 and 95 per cent of sufferers of both are women. Thus the two disorders show a number of similarities. Nevertheless, the two are sufficiently distinct to be worthy of separate examination (Mussell *et al.* 2000). For both these eating disorders we consider definitions, causal factors and common treatments. It is widely accepted that eating disorders are multifactorially determined, with sociocultural, biological and psychological factors contributing to their development (Kaye *et al.* 2000). Among the psychological variables implicated are depression, low self-esteem, body dissatisfaction, lack of assertiveness and psychological distress (Ball and Lee 1999). As we noted earlier, such body dissatisfaction in women is probably linked to social pressures towards attaining unattainably slim body shapes.

Anorexia nervosa

Anorexia nervosa is an eating disorder characterized by 'the relentless pursuit of thinness through self-starvation, even unto death' (Bruch 1973: 3). It is a disorder that principally affects females in their mid to late teens. Only about 10 per cent of anorexics are male. Anorexics tend to be white and from upper-middle or upper class backgrounds. Crisp *et al.* (1976) report prevalence rates of approximately 1 per cent in schoolgirls aged 16 years or over in private schools and about 0.2 per cent in state schools. Although community studies report that around 5 per cent of young women show some, but not all, of the features of anorexia (Szmukler 1989), the rate in the general female population is estimated to be 0.3–0.7 per cent (Kaye *et al.* 2000).

The characteristics of anorexia include a lack of food intake, but *without* a corresponding loss of appetite. Indeed, anorexics are frequently reported to be obsessed with food and food consumption. In addition, to be diagnosed as anorexic, the individual must be at least 15 per cent below his or her minimum normal body weight for height. In women, diagnosis also involves the cessation of menstruating.

The most common clinical history involves the commencement of a diet aimed at improving body shape (Szmukler 1989). Despite increasing weight loss the individual continues to restrict her food intake. Food and body weight become major preoccupations. In the restricting subtype of anorexia, simple self-starvation is principally employed to reduce or maintain a below normal body weight. The binge eating/purging subtype is also characterized by episodes of binge eating, usually combined with a compensatory strategy such as induced vomiting and the use of large quantities of laxatives. Another common symptom of anorexia is excessive exercise, often of a strenuous nature and for several hours each day, all in the pursuit of further weight loss. Anorexics have an intense fear of becoming 'fat', which does not appear to diminish with weight loss. Those treating anorexics frequently report that a striking feature is the denial of thinness even in the face of extreme emaciation (Szmukler 1989). They often report an unrelenting obsession with fatness along with an inexplicable fear of weight gain (Kaye *et al.* 2000).

A large number of factors have been suggested as causes of anorexia. No one factor has yet emerged as a dominant or indeed sufficient cause. Most researchers now consider that anorexia is best viewed as being multiply determined. Some authors have argued that societal pressure for a thin ideal body shape for women (noted earlier) has been a major factor in the apparently increased incidence of the disorder. This explanation is in accord with the observed increasingly thin ideal body image and increasing levels of anorexia observed in the latter part of the twentieth century. It is also consistent with reports that such pressures are greater and the incidence of anorexia is higher in particular groups, such as women generally or those attending ballet schools more specifically (Szmukler 1989). Some authors argue that anorexia and other eating disorders should be conceptualized as the extreme end of the continuum of bodily concern and dieting, rather than as a specific clinical group (Charles and Kerr 1986; Chesters 1994;

Grogan and Cortvreind submitted). However, it seems unlikely that such pressures alone are sufficient to cause anorexia (Kaye *et al.* 2000). What such pressures may do is increase levels of dieting (in order to achieve desired body shapes), and that dieting exposes more vulnerable individuals to the possible development of anorexia.

There is increasing evidence of a genetic basis to anorexia. For example, Holland *et al.* (1984) report a higher concordance rate for anorexia in monozygotic twins (55 per cent) than in dizygotic twins (7 per cent). More recent research has focused on physiological differences in the neuroendocrine system, including differences in neuropeptides and serotonin, as potential determinants of anorexia (Kaye *et al.* 2000).

Psychological factors also appear to be important for understanding anorexia. Some of these factors focus on the other functions that the behaviours associated with the disorder may fulfil. For example, many anorexics are seen as using anorexia as a way of dealing with various life problems. The behaviours associated with anorexia may be used as a way of gaining attention, as an attempt at asserting individuality, as a denial of sexuality or as a resolution to the problems of dealing with overdemanding parents. A common theme is the idea that restricting food intake is a way of exerting control (Orbach 1993). Nevertheless, anorexics generally appear not to recognize the harm that the food restriction is causing them and not to be able to explain their own behaviour fully (Szmukler 1989). It has proved difficult to research the determinants of anorexia because of difficulties in recruiting adequate prospective samples because of the young age of onset. Thus much research in this area relies on comparison of those with the disorder and those who recover from the disorder. Bruch (1973) proposed that underlying anorexia are a number of specific disturbances, including disturbance of body image, difficulties identifying internal sensations and a sense of personal ineffectiveness.

Anorexics appear to have negative attitudes towards their own body shape and show distorted perceptions of it. The latter has received particular attention. In general, anorexics tend to see themselves as heavier than they really are. A variety of techniques for measuring accurate perception of body size have been developed (Garfinkel and Garner 1982). Although there is considerable variation across studies, there appears to be a general tendency for anorexics to overestimate their body size compared to controls. For example, Garner *et al.* (1980) used a distorting photograph technique to demonstrate this tendency compared to normal weight respondents. Interestingly, this biased tendency did not extend to anorexics' estimation of the body shape of others, suggesting the bias is specific to their view of themselves rather than an aspect of the way they view the world. Interestingly, it is not clear that this overestimation of one's own body shape is more extreme in anorexic compared to simply thin women (see Grogan 1999).

The evidence concerning changes in the perception and interpretation of internal stimuli such as hunger and satiety is even less clear-cut. While studies have demonstrated that anorexics report a general lack of hunger and feelings of satiation after consuming very small quantities of food (e.g. Owen *et al.* 1985), it is not clear whether these are a cause or a consequence of self-starvation. More consistent evidence relates to distinct personality traits, such as perfectionism, conformity, obsessionality, restrained emotional expressiveness and reduced social spontaneity (Kaye *et al.* 2000). It is interesting to note that such traits appear before the onset of illness and persist even after long-term weight recovery. This would suggest that they are not merely the result of the disordered eating but are more fundamental to the development of the disorder. Stress is another factor linked to the onset of anorexia (Ball and Lee 1999), and is considered in more detail in Chapter 5.

Van Buskirk (1977) distinguishes two groups of treatment for anorexia. It is generally agreed that psychotherapeutic interventions are unlikely to be helpful while the individual is emaciated. Therefore, the first group of treatments focus on producing rapid weight gain in dangerously underweight anorexics, occasionally without the individual's consent. These include forced feeding, drug therapy and behaviour therapy. For example, behaviour therapy typically involves making the performance of valued activities contingent on eating or weight gain. This usually requires inpatient treatment within a hospital setting over a period of 6–12 weeks (Szmukler 1989). Drug treatment appears to have a limited role at this stage.

The second group of treatments focus on maintaining or prolonging weight gain over a greater period of time and usually take place in an outpatient setting. Unfortunately, weight restoration appears to be more easily achieved than weight maintenance, with 30–50 per cent of anorexics requiring readmission to hospital because of subsequent weight loss (Szmukler 1989). The techniques used at this stage include individual, group and family therapy, and self-help groups (Bruch 1973; Garner and Bemis 1982). For example, cognitive–behaviour therapy uses principles derived from learning theory to modify the patient's thoughts and feelings about eating. Russell *et al.* (1987) have shown that family therapy, where the family is the focus of the psychotherapy, was more effective than individual therapy for those with an early onset of the illness. This suggests an important role for dysfunctional family relationships, at least in the development of early onset anorexia. Despite these encouraging findings, there is currently a lack of well designed controlled studies on the long-term effectiveness of treatments for anorexia.

Recovery from anorexia is a long-term process. Few anorexics recover in less than two years, while about one-third do within three years. Beyond four years the rate of recovery tails off. Overall complete recovery rates are reported to be around 50 per cent, while a further 30 per cent experience lingering problems. A further 10 per cent have chronic, unremitting problems, while the remaining 10 per cent will eventually die from anorexia (Kaye *et al.* 2000). Poorer outcomes are predicted by older age of onset, longer duration of illness and lower body weight at admission to hospital.

Bulimia nervosa

Bulimia nervosa is defined as recurrent binge eating accompanied by a feeling of lack of control over eating, followed by purging, and a persistent over-concern with body shape and weight (American Psychiatric Association 1994). Bulimia usually emerges after a period of dieting, which may or may not have resulted in weight loss (Kaye *et al.* 2000). The binges appear to be a loss of control over the restriction of food intake. They tend to be intermittent and only develop some time after the individual starts to restrict food intake. The binges typically consist of the consumption of a large amount of food in a discrete period of time. They typically occur once per day, frequently in the evening, and consist of consuming an average of 4800 calories, usually in the form of sweet or salty foods high in carbohydrate (Johnson-Sabine *et al.* 1982). Thus the average binge involves consuming roughly twice the daily intake of food in a single eating session. The purging can take various forms, including self-induced vomiting and the use of laxatives or diuretics. In Johnson-Sabine *et al.*'s study, 81 per cent regularly purged using self-induced vomiting and 63 per cent regularly used laxatives. A non-purging type of bulimia reacts to binges with other compensatory acts, such as strict dieting or excessive vigorous exercise. The majority of bulimics maintain a weight that is within the normal range, although the bingeing and purging can have serious physiological effects. These include sore throats, poor dental health, dehydration, cardiac arrhythmias, urinary problems and even epileptic seizures.

Bulimics tend to be women in their late teens or early twenties. The binge episodes tend to produce high levels of distress. Preoccupations with food and weight can be extremely disruptive to the individual's daily life and the amount of money spent on food can be exorbitant (Szmukler 1989). The incidence rate is between 1.7 and 2.5 per cent (Kaye *et al.* 2000), although more than 50 per cent of women in some surveys report at least some symptoms of bulimia (Szmukler 1989). Follow-up studies indicate that around 50 per cent of bulimics recovered between five and ten years after diagnosis, while between 20 and 30 per cent still meet the classification criteria even after this prolonged period of time.

Similarly to anorexia, a number of possible causes of bulimia have been suggested. Twin studies suggest that there may be a genetic basis to bulimia (Kaye *et al.* 2000). Bulimics also tend to be dissatisfied with their body image, wanting to be smaller than they currently are and having a low ideal body weight. Stice (1994) argues that bulimics internalize the unrealistic ideal body weight presented in Western societies, resulting in body dissatisfaction. In turn the body dissatisfaction leads to dietary restraint and so increases the chances of binge eating and bulimia in those with other predisposing characteristics. The bingeing episodes have been interpreted as fulfilling some emotional need, because they seem to be more likely following certain social situations and stressful events. There is also some evidence to suggest that bulimia is an extreme form of restraint. Restrained eaters tend to restrict their food intake, but respond to a preload of food by breaking this restraint and consuming more rather than less food (Herman 1978). Bulimics are also preoccupied with food and obsessed with limiting food intake between binges. Similarly, bulimics often report a similar pattern to their food intake to restrained individuals, with their usual restraint being broken by a binge brought on by eating a small amount of a 'forbidden' food, drinking alcohol or feeling depressed (Szmukler 1989). It has been suggested that depression is an additional causal factor in bulimia.

Behaviour therapy and cognitive–behaviour therapy are commonly employed to treat bulimia. Cognitive–behaviour therapy, in particular, appears to be effective for at least 60–70 per cent of individuals and improves symptoms such as body dissatisfaction, pursuit of thinness and perfectionism (Kaye *et al.* 2000). In addition, exposure and response prevention, where the patient is exposed to the anxiety that accompanies excessive food intake without purging, is commonly employed. The combined use of cognitive–behaviour therapy with exposure and response prevention has also produced long-term reductions in bingeing and purging. In addition, several studies report that anti-depressants are effective in treating bulimia (Pope *et al.* 1983). However, the effectiveness of anti-depressants may diminish over time and they do not appear to add to the effectiveness of psychotherapy.

Summary

This chapter reviewed research on weight control and disorders of eating. Issues of weight control are important for both health and aesthetic reasons. Deviations from normal weight are associated with various health problems, which increase in severity and likelihood the more extreme are the deviations. In Westernized nations with ready access to an abundant, palatable food supply, excess weight is much more of a problem than too low a weight. Weight control is also an important issue because of the high value placed upon particular (slim) body shapes. Social psychologists have made important contributions to the understanding of this latter issue. Extreme overweight or obesity is caused by a range of factors, including genetic and behavioural factors. A variety of methods have been employed to control weight. These can be generally grouped into reducing energy intake or increasing energy expenditure. A number of these strategies are efficacious in reducing weight but have been shown to be of limited value in maintaining weight loss. Advances in our understanding of the basis of the maintenance of weight control behaviours may lead on to effective interventions for maintaining weight loss. The final part of the chapter reviewed the ways in which our understanding of the serious eating disorders anorexia and bulimia nervosa have increased in recent years.

Suggested further reading

Brownell, K.D. and Wadden, T.A. (1992) Etiology and treatment of obesity: Understanding a serious, prevalent, and refactory disorder, *Journal of Consulting and Clinical Psychology*, 60: 505–17.

A broad review of the causes and treatment of a major disorder.

Grogan, S. (1999) *Body Image: Understanding Body Dissatisfaction in Men, Women and Children*. London: Routledge.

This book provides a useful overview of research on body image and the social psychological research on body dissatisfaction.

Woods, S.C., Schwartz, M.W., Baskin, D.G. and Seeley, R.J. (2000) Food intake and the regulation of body weight, *Annual Review of Psychology*, 51: 255–77.

A comprehensive review of research on the relationship between food intake and body weight control processes.

5

Stress and eating

General overview

The study of stress and its effects has occupied the attention of a large number of researchers from a variety of disciplines, including psychology. One important effect of stress that has been noted is the impact on eating behaviour. While much of the psychological research in this area has started from a physiological perspective, recent work has begun to highlight the importance of social psychological variables such as attitudes in influencing the relationship of stress to eating. The present chapter provides a review of this broader literature and then moves on to consider some of the interesting questions on stress–eating relationships that this work poses for social psychologists. The chapter begins with a review of how stress has been defined and the general implications for eating. The next section briefly reviews work on the general effect of stress on eating. The major section of the chapter then reviews the individual difference approach to stress–eating relationships. This approach suggests that stress produces different effects (increased, decreased or no change) on eating in different groups. The major groups considered are the obese versus the non-obese, the restrained (i.e. dieter) versus the non-restrained and men versus women. Two other groupings that have received less attention are those high versus low in emotional or external eating. In the next section we consider what research has taught us about the impact of stress on disordered eating. The final section considers a number of social psychological questions that this research poses. In particular, issues concerning the type and severity of the stress, which groups are affected, the types of food affected and the potential mechanisms are considered.

Definitions of stress and implications for eating

The concept of stress has proved very difficult to define and operationalize. However, it is generally agreed that stress is an aversive state in which the well-being of the organism is threatened, and it is commonly assumed to be the result of the individual's perception that the demands of the environment exceed, or threaten to exceed, the available resources to cope (Lazarus and Folkman 1984). Stress has been examined in both experimental and correlational research. In experimental research, stressors include mood manipulations (e.g. videos of unpleasant accidents), cognitive tasks (e.g. counting backward by sevens) and physical stressors (e.g. partial immersion in very cold water) presented in the laboratory. Such manipulations have the clear advantage of ensuring that each participant is exposed to the same stressor. However, such stressors are generally weaker and of shorter duration than those experienced in naturalistic settings (e.g. death of a close relative).

In correlational research, the key issue has been how to define and measure stressors. Early approaches focused on stressful major life events, such as bereavement, divorce or job loss (e.g. Holmes and Rahe 1967). Later work has emphasized the stressful nature of many minor life events, often referred to as hassles (Delongis *et al.* 1984). These include irritating, but minor, events, such as losing one's keys. Both these approaches to examining the effects of stress share disadvantages. It may be that an event defined as stressful has quite different *characteristics* for different individuals. For example, job loss might remove one's principal source of income and require a considerable period of time and perhaps retraining before another job can be found. Alternatively, the loss of income resulting from job loss might be offset by redundancy payments and the finding of an alternative, more attractive job. Similarly, the same event might be *perceived* quite differently: job loss could be seen as a threat to a view of oneself as a useful member of a family, community or society; alternatively it could be seen as a release from a difficult, boring and generally unrewarding situation. Hence, another approach taken in this area to counteract these problems is to assess self-reported level of stress (i.e. perceived stress; Cohen *et al.* 1983). While obviating the above problems, this approach clearly introduces new problems concerning the reliability and validity of self-report measures.

As the above paragraphs make clear, there is no one widely accepted approach to defining and studying stress and its effects. Nevertheless, the differing approaches can usefully complement one another. Together these approaches have provided a number of important insights into the relationship between stress and health.

In a review of work on these different measures of stress and eating behaviour, Greeno and Wing (1994) suggested that two general hypotheses have been investigated: first, a *general effect hypothesis* that stress changes consumption of food generally; second, an *individual difference hypothesis* that stress leads to changes in eating in particular groups (e.g. the obese, restrained eaters, women). It is this work we now go on to review.

The general effect of stress on eating

The majority of early work on stress–eating relationships investigated the so-called 'general effect model' (Figure 5.1). It is assumed that stress produces a general response to eating. Such a model is particularly consistent with stress producing physiological changes in the organism and these changes explaining changes in eating behaviour. Research in this paradigm has particularly focused on animal research. So, for example, Antelman *et al.* (1975) induced stress in rats by pinching their tails and observed significant increases in gnawing, eating and licking of food. Other such studies have used electric shocks and cold water as stressors, while further studies have used chronic stressors such as isolation (Robbins and Fray 1980; Greeno and Wing 1994). In general this research provides some support for the general effect model of stress, although the effects are not wholly consistent. While tail-pinching does appear generally to increase oral behaviours, including eating, it is not clear that this represents stress-induced eating. There is less evidence for effects of other stressors (e.g. electric shock, cold water), although the chronic stressor of isolation does appear consistently to increase eating and weight in rats (Greeno and Wing 1994). What is less clear is whether this effect is peculiar to isolation or general to all chronic stressors. Further work of this nature with other chronic stressors is required to answer these questions.

Similarly, the few published human studies testing the general effect model have produced mixed results. Bellisle *et al.* (1990) found no evidence that an acute stressor changed the amount or type of foods eaten in a group of men. The amount and types of food eaten by a group of men on the morning before they were to undergo surgery was compared with a later day when they were not due to undergo surgery. However, both testing situations took place in the hospital where surgery was undergone, and this in itself might have produced moderately high levels of stress on both occasions, masking the stress–eating relationship. In contrast, Michaud *et al.* (1990) found the stress of an impending examination to increase calorie intake, particularly from fatty foods such as snacks, in a sample of school children. In general, all children were found to eat more on examination compared to non-examination days and in particular to eat more fatty foods, although the differences between days were only significant for girls.

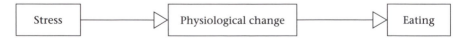

Figure 5.1   The general effect model of the stress–eating relationship

Hence, in summary, research on the general effects model indicates that stress generally produces an increase in food intake. However, the evidence is principally from animal studies and by no means overwhelming. In addition, it is not yet clear whether the type of stressor (acute versus chronic) is important. Finally, the mechanisms by which stress influences eating in the general effect model remain underinvestigated.

The individual difference approach to stress–eating relationships

The individual difference model of stress–eating relationships (Figure 5.2) suggests that differences in learning history, attitudes towards eating or biology produce variations in vulnerability to the effects of stress. Those exhibiting vulnerability respond to stress with an environmental or psychological change that promotes eating. In contrast, those with low vulnerability exhibit a different environmental or psychological change that does not promote eating. The precise nature of these mechanisms has been less investigated. We will return to consider psychological mechanisms later in the chapter.

Individual difference models predict that groups reflecting different levels of vulnerability will differ in their eating behaviour when stressed. Several such groups have been proposed, and relevant research is examined below. These groups include differences between: the obese and non-obese; the restrained (i.e. those attempting to control their food intake or dieters) and unrestrained; women and men; emotional and non-emotional eaters; external and internal eaters. It should be clear that the proposed mechanisms relating stress to eating in the general effect and individual difference approaches are different. The general effect approach principally assumes that stress produces a physiological/biological change that in turn causes a change in eating. In contrast, the individual difference approach tends to posit psychological or environmental mechanisms to explain the changes in eating in the different groups. Some of these proposed mechanisms are touched upon below.

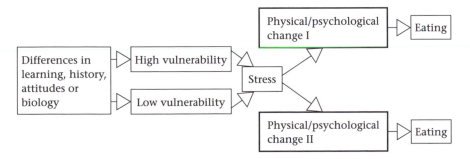

Figure 5.2   The individual difference model of the stress–eating relationship

Obese versus non-obese

Initial interest in the effect of stress on eating in humans began as an attempt to understand obesity. It was suggested that overweight individuals were more likely to respond to stressful or emotional stimuli by eating (Stunkard 1959). Such views arose from psychosomatic views of obesity, which suggested that obese individuals did not learn to distinguish between hunger and anxiety (Kaplan and Kaplan 1957). Such individuals were assumed to respond to stress as if it were hunger (i.e. by eating). An alternative view was put forward by Schachter *et al.* (1968). These researchers suggested that unlike normal weight individuals, obese individuals had not learned to label various physiological cues (e.g. gastric contractions) as hunger. It was suggested that these cues reduce under stress. Therefore the prediction was that stress should produce a reduction in hunger and eating in normal weight individuals but have no impact on the feelings of hunger and eating behaviour in the obese. Thus the two accounts both predict differences in eating behaviour of the obese and non-obese in response to stress. However, the direction of change is different in the two accounts. In the Schachter *et al.* account it was predicted that stress would *decrease* eating in normal weight individuals and have no effect on obese individuals. The psychosomatic account predicted stress to *increase* eating in obese individuals and have no effect on normal weight individuals. The evidence for these different predictions is reviewed separately.

Greeno and Wing (1994) reviewed 11 studies that addressed the effect of stress on eating in obese and non-obese groups. Schachter *et al.* (1968) produced the first laboratory test of this effect. Anticipating a painful compared to a mild shock (high versus low stress) produced a decrease in eating in normal weight participants, but had no effect on obese participants. This finding is consistent with the Schachter *et al.* model just outlined. However, only one of the other ten tests of this hypothesis reviewed by Greeno and Wing (1994) produced a similar decrease in consumption in normal weight individuals. The other studies generally observed no change in consumption in response to stress in normal weight individuals. This represents very weak support for the Schachter *et al.* account of the impact of stress on eating in non-obese groups.

The support for the psychosomatic account has also been reported to be mixed. Of the 11 studies reviewed by Greeno and Wing (1994), three demonstrated an increase in eating for obese individuals when stressed, three found that some obese individuals eat more when stressed, but five further studies failed to find a relationship between stress and eating in obese individuals. Taken together this is only relatively modest support for the psychosomatic account of stress–eating relationships in the obese. In addition, those studies only finding partial support for the psychosomatic account suggest an alternative view of these relationships. For example, Baucom and Aiken (1981) demonstrated that it was dieting rather than obesity that was the key predictor of stress-related eating in their study. For both obese and non-obese groups, stress only produced increases in eating in the dieting group. Given the fact that many obese individuals are dieting in an attempt to control their weight, the failure to control for dieting may explain the contradictory findings across studies on the impacts of stress on eating in the obese. In effect, it may be that because dieting is more prevalent in the obese than the non-obese this explains why stress leads to greater eating in the obese compared to the non-obese group.

Restrained versus unrestrained

The concept of restrained eating developed from the 'set point' theory of obesity (Herman and Polivy 1975; see Chapter 4). Restrained eaters are assumed to restrict their food intake through self-control processes. When these self-control processes are undermined, disinhibition of eating occurs, and excessive food intake takes place. For example, restrained eaters appear not to adjust their food intake for previous food intake (Herman and Mack 1975). Unrestrained eaters adjust for consuming a 'preload' of food by eating less in a subsequent eating test; restrained eaters do not appear to perform this adjustment and eat just as much as if they had not eaten the preload. It is believed that the preload disinhibits the restraint over eating they normally show. Stress is also expected to affect restrained eaters by disrupting the control that they normally try to exert over their eating. Thus, individuals with high restraint scores should be more likely to respond to stress by eating, while those low in restraint should show no change. Heatherton *et al.* (1991) and Schotte *et al.* (1990) both compared high- and low-restrained eaters, and found that not only did restrained women eat more than unrestrained women, but restrained women who were stressed ate more than restrained women who were not stressed. Cools *et al.* (1992) used restraint as a continuous variable, rather than dividing subjects into high- and low-restraint groups, and showed that the stressed group consumed progressively more food as restraint scores increased. A number of other studies reviewed by Greeno and Wing (1994) also generally produce consistent results: stress produced greater increase in eating in restrained compared to unrestrained eaters. Nevertheless, it must be conceded that the vast majority of studies to date have only demonstrated this effect in college-aged women. Future research needs to confirm these effects in other samples (i.e. non-college samples, men). Wardle *et al.* (2000) showed that work stress led to increased eating in restrained women and men. The effect of restraint in men is an issue that is particularly worthy of further study.

Women versus men

Several studies have looked at differences in female versus male eating in response to stress. Grunberg and Straub (1992) looked at whether there are differences between women and men in vulnerability to what they called 'stress-induced eating' (i.e. eating more when stressed than not stressed). Sweet, salty and bland foods were provided for subjects while they were watching a video, and for half the subjects the video was unpleasant (i.e. stress inducing). Results showed that unstressed men consumed significantly more food than any other group. However, stressed women consumed twice as much sweet food as unstressed women, suggesting the importance of food type, at least in women. Although stress generally reduced eating in men, this effect was not significant. Pine (1985) compared obese and non-obese men and women, and found that stress-induced eating was more pronounced among women than among men. Stone and Brownell (1994) examined the relationship between stress and eating for married couples, who completed daily records of stress and eating. Results showed that both men and women were likely to eat less than usual in response to stress, and the tendency to eat less with an increasing severity of stress was particularly pronounced in women. It is not clear why increased levels of stress were associated with decreased rather than increased eating in this sample.

Thus the evidence for gender differences in stress-induced eating is somewhat contradictory. The effects appear to be generally greater in women than men, but some studies report stress to increase eating, others to decrease eating and yet others to have no effect on eating. Some of the effects also appear to be peculiar to particular types of food (e.g. sweet foods). Interpretation of these findings is further complicated by the fact that gender is found to be correlated with restrained eating (i.e. women generally show higher levels of restraint). In addition, very few studies have examined the effect of restraint on stress–eating relationships in men.

Emotional versus non-emotional eaters

Emotional eating refers to a tendency to eat more when anxious or emotionally aroused compared to non-emotional eaters, who do not show such reactivity to emotion in their eating habits. Emotional eating is found to be generally higher in women than men (van Strein *et al.* 1986). Stress is assumed to lead to increased eating in emotional eaters because they fail to distinguish between anxiety and hunger (i.e. they respond to stress as if it were hunger), while not affecting those low in emotional eating. The origins in psychosomatic approaches to understanding stress–eating relationships discussed above in relation to obesity should be clear. Psychometric measures of emotional eating have been developed (e.g. van Strein *et al.* 1986). Van Strein and colleagues found that stressful life events predicted weight gain in men over a period of 18 months, but only among those who were emotional eaters. In women, stress led to weight gain irrespective of their level of emotional eating. Other studies have reported limited impact (Schlundt *et al.* 1991) or a lack of impact (e.g. Conner *et al.* 1999) of emotional eating on stress–eating relationships. Given the limited number of published studies of emotional eating, its impact on stress–eating relationships remains an issue for further study.

Summary of research on the individual difference approach to stress–eating relationships

As the above review of research makes clear, the individual difference approach to stress–eating relationships has raised as many issues as it has answered. Normal weight individuals appear to be generally unaffected by stress in terms of their eating. Obese individuals show mixed reactions to stress in terms of their eating behaviour. Greeno and Wing (1994) suggest that the findings are almost equally divided between suggesting that stress increases, decreases or has no effect on eating in obese groups. In contrast, restrained young women, when exposed to laboratory stressors, tend to increase their food intake. The greater levels of restraint in women might account for the fact that stress-induced eating is more common in women than men. Finally, there is limited support for the idea that those who identify themselves as emotional eaters are more likely to engage in stress-induced eating.

One interesting fact about the above studies on the individual difference approach to stress–eating relationships is the failure to examine these individual difference variables simultaneously. This is surprising given the relationship between variables. For example, restrained eaters are reported to be more likely also to be emotional eaters (Weissenburger *et al.* 1986) and external eaters (Heatherton and Baumeister 1991; see below). We have already noted the relationship of gender to emotional and restrained eating. Research examining such variables simultaneously would allow us more accurately to compare the relative effects of these individual difference variables. One study that has attempted to do this is the study by Conner *et al.* (1999), which we will examine in a little more detail than other research reviewed here.

The study of Conner *et al.* (1999) was concerned with whether the number of daily stressors (hassles) affect eating behaviour (snacking), and whether external eating, emotional eating, restrained eating, gender or severity of stress moderate this relationship. Based on a review of the literature, the authors expected snacking to be used by respondents as a way of coping with stress (Lazarus and Folkman 1984), and this coping mechanism to be more employed by particular groups (women, external, emotional and restrained eaters). To investigate these relationships, a seven-day diary method was used because it allowed the authors to examine these interrelationships in everyday life. Between-meal snacks were selected as the measure of eating because this is a discrete form of eating commonly reported as a response to stress (Warr and Payne 1982; Spillman 1990; Zerbe 1993). It is also likely to be accurately reported, but had not been a focus of many previous studies. Snacking is also of interest because it is a behaviour perceived to lead to problems with weight control (Conner and Norman 1996; Grogan *et al.* 1997). The use of an open-ended diary allowed respondents to record what snacks were consumed each day and avoided problems of memory lapse over longer periods, which are common when individuals are asked to recall relatively mundane behaviours (Conner and Waterman 1996). Diaries are similarly appropriate for recording instances of stressful events (Verbrugge 1984; Wheeler and Reis 1991). The stressful events recorded were minor life events or hassles. Hassles are daily stressors, and can be defined as problems or difficulties that are part of everyday life. Hassles are events, thoughts or situations which, when they occur, produce negative feelings such as annoyance, irritation, worry or frustration, and/or make you aware that your goals and plans will be more difficult or impossible to achieve. Hassles occur more frequently than, for example, major life events, and occur for most people. Thus, measuring hassles allowed quite a large number of stress occurrences in each respondent to be identified, making it possible to look at whether snacking coincided with hassles on a number of occasions. This would then provide a good test of whether eating changed in response to stress. Like other researchers looking at the impact of stress on eating (e.g. Stone and Brownell 1994), Conner *et al.* employed an open-ended measure of hassles that allowed respondents to write in the events they found stressful. Such measures have the advantage of not constraining respondents to a limited number of events. In addition, respondents were required to indicate the severity of each hassle as experienced. This can be regarded as a measure of perceived stress, referred to at the beginning of this chapter. This was used as another individual difference variable to examine if severity of stress influenced the general stress (number of hassles experienced) to eating (number of snacks consumed) relationship.

Interestingly, Conner *et al.* (1999) also examined both men and women and three other individual difference variables thought to influence stress–eating relationships. These three variables were restrained, emotional and external eating and were assessed by self-report questionnaire (van Strien *et al.* 1986). Restrained eating was assessed by items such as 'When you have put on weight, do you eat less than you usually do?' Emotional eating was assessed by items such as 'Do you have a desire to eat when you are irritated?' Finally, the measure of external eating was based upon 'externality theory' (Schachter *et al.* 1968), which suggests that external eaters eat in response to food-related stimuli, regardless of the internal state of hunger and satiety, while internal eaters are more responsive to internal cues such as hunger in deciding to eat. This was assessed by items such as 'If food tastes good to you, do you eat more than usual?' (all items responded to on 'never–very often' scales).

The overall results indicated that on average the sample consumed 1.4 snacks per day and reported approximately one hassle per day (which was rated as between 'somewhat' and 'quite a bit' of a problem in terms of severity). Number of snacks was significantly positively correlated with number of hassles. Thus for days when respondents reported greater numbers of hassles they also reported consuming more snacks compared to days for which they reported few hassles. Thus, Conner *et al.* demonstrate a general relationship between stress and eating (i.e. a greater number of experienced hassles is related to a greater consumption of snacks). This finding is in direct contrast to the findings of Stone and Brownell (1994), who, using a similar methodology, reported stress being more consistently related to eating less (72 per cent of consistent respondents) than eating more (28 per cent of consistent respondents). However, a major difference between the two studies is the dependent variable, which was eating more or less generally in the Stone and Brownell study, and number of snacks consumed in the Conner *et al.* study. It may well be that eating more snacks is associated with a general reduction in the amount eaten or amount perceived to be eaten, through breaking up the pattern of meals eaten. This might usefully be investigated in future studies. The Conner *et al.* findings suggest that stress might increase the consumption of snacks. This might be important no matter what the effect on general eating patterns because of the suggestion that between-meal snacking can lead to problems of weight control (Conner and Norman 1996; Grogan *et al.* 1997).

Subsequent analyses of the Conner *et al.* study examined the extent to which severity of stress, gender, restraint, emotional eating or external eating influenced this relationship between stress and eating. Severity of hassles did not have any effect on the relationship between hassles and snacking; for hassles perceived to be severe or not severe, more hassles were associated with consuming more snacks. For gender, there was a non-significant effect of hassles on snacking for men, but a significant effect for women, although the difference between the two was not statistically significant. Nevertheless, this would appear to provide some support for other literature which suggests that stress–eating relationships are stronger in women. In relation to restrained and emotional eating, there was no evidence of an impact on the stress–eating relationship; increasing hassles were associated with eating more snacks at both high and low levels of these two variables. In contrast, external eating did show evidence of moderation of the relationship between hassles and snacks. This suggests a different relationship between hassles and snacking at different levels of external eating. The precise nature of this moderation effect was investigated by plotting the regression lines of number of snacks on number of hassles at the mean level of external eating and at low and high levels of external eating (Figure 5.3). At low levels of external eating there is a non-significant negative impact of number of hassles on number of snacks consumed. However, at high levels of external eating the relationship is a significant positive one, indicating that higher levels of hassles were associated with higher levels of snacking. These results partially support the Schachterian/externality theory on which the external eating scale is based (van Strien *et al.* 1986). Externality theory proposes that eating in external eaters decreases in response to stress. Conner *et al.*'s data revealed such a negative relationship, although it was not statistically significant. The definition of external eating used by van Strien *et al.* (1986: 296) is 'eating in

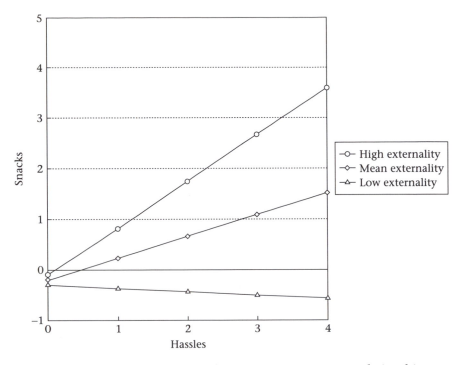

Figure 5.3 The impact of external eating on stress–eating relationships
Source: from Conner *et al.* 1999.

response to food related stimuli, regardless of the internal state of hunger and satiety'. However, since stress has also been shown to draw attention to external cues (e.g. Heatherton and Baumeister 1991), one might expect stress to lead to increased eating in external eaters by making (external) cues to eating more salient, while having no impact upon non-external eaters. This might explain the increase in eating in response to stress observed in the high external eating group by Conner *et al.* This is similar to the explanation of stress-induced eating in animals provided by Robbins and Fray (1980). Stressors are assumed to increase anxiety and make organisms more responsive to external stimuli in their eating. Organisms then eat more because they have difficulty discriminating between the internal stimuli of anxiety or hunger. The data of Conner *et al.* suggest that this is particularly true for individuals high on the construct of externality. It is interesting that it is externality that emerged as the individual difference variable that produced variations in stress–eating relationships. Further studies, replicating the findings of Conner *et al.*, and examining several of the proposed individual difference variables simultaneously, are required before we place too much reliance on the finding that externality is the key moderator of stress–eating relationships.

The results of the Conner *et al.* study show that some groups are more likely to respond to stress by eating – those high on external eating show stronger positive hassles–snacking relationships – while others are less likely to respond to stress by eating – those low on external eating show no hassles – snacking relationships. Snacking may be seen as an attempt at coping with the stressor (Lazarus and Folkman 1984). Heatherton and Baumeister (1991) argue that stress-induced eating helps individuals to escape distress by focusing on external stimuli. This explanation seems to apply particularly well to external eaters. Since external eaters rely on food-related stimuli to trigger eating, and not the internal hunger state, it seems viable that over-awareness of food cues is likely to increase when under stress, since stress has been shown to focus attention on external stimuli. Increased over-awareness of food cues might force the individual to focus on the immediate situation and avoid meaningful thought about the problem. Food consumption would thus be likely to increase, since external eaters rely on these cues to trigger eating, and so eating in external eaters could be seen as a coping attempt. Conner *et al.* also examined whether there were further moderation effects among variables (e.g. did restraint moderate stress–eating relationships just in women?). However, no evidence was found for such effects.

The impact of stress on disordered eating

The above work has focused on the relationship between stress and eating in non-eating disordered populations. There is, however, also a large literature on the impacts of stress on the development of disordered eating, which we briefly review here (see Ball and Lee 1999).

As noted in Chapter 4, eating disorders such as anorexia, bulimia and binge eating have serious medical and psychological consequences (French and Jeffery 1994). It is widely accepted that such disorders are determined by multiple factors, including sociocultural, biological and psychological influences. Among the psychological factors considered to be important are depression, low self-esteem and body esteem and lack of assertiveness. In addition, psychological stress appears to show relatively consistent relationships with disordered eating (Ball and Lee 1999). Ball and Lee provide a useful review of this literature and examine the impacts of stress assessed both by life event measures and by perceived stress. In both literatures, the majority of studies report a consistent relationship between stress and disordered eating; increasing levels of stress are found to be associated with an increasing incidence of disordered eating. This was true for studies of anorexics (Crisp *et al.* 1980), bulimics (Lacey *et al.* 1986) and binge eaters (Hawkins and Clement 1980) with respect to life event measures of stress. Similar patterns were found for anorexics (Haslam *et al.* 1989) and bulimics/binge eaters (Crowther and Chernyk 1986) using a measure of perceived stress. Hence, there appears to be good evidence of an association between stress and disordered eating.

However, closer examination of these studies indicates that the vast majority of studies were cross-sectional, with measures of stress and disordered eating taken at the same time point. Such data do not allow us to distinguish clearly between the impact of stress on disordered eating and the impact of disordered eating on stress (i.e. the direction of causation is unclear). This problem is additional to other concerns with inferring causation from correlational evidence (e.g. third variables causing both variables). Of the studies reviewed by Ball and Lee (1999), only two employed prospective designs (Rosen *et al.* 1990, 1993). What was interesting in these two studies was that although a significant relationship was observed between a life event measure of stress and disordered eating, the direction of effect appeared to be from disordered eating to stress. Thus it may be that disordered eating leads to an increased probability of certain life events (e.g. by producing disruptions in social/family relationships). This explanation of stress-disordered eating relationships requires further study.

Thus, while research on the relationship between stress and disordered eating appears to indicate a fairly robust coexistence of the two variables, the evidence that stress promotes disordered eating is weaker. Indeed, the few available studies looking at how the relationships between these two variables unfold over time would appear to be more supportive of the view that disordered eating leads to higher levels of stress. Further research is required to examine the causal direction of the relationship between stress and disordered eating and the potential mechanisms underlying this relationship.

Future directions for research on stress–eating relationships

The research reviewed in this chapter suggests that there is no simple relationship between stress and eating. Only very limited evidence, mainly in animal studies, exists to support the idea that stress produces a general change in eating. However, it does appear that stress can produce different effects on eating in different groups. Nevertheless, considerably more work is required to provide further insights into these relationships. Key issues revolve around the nature of the stress, the nature of the eating behaviour, the groups likely to be affected and the possible mechanisms of effect. Each of these issues is briefly considered in this section.

The nature of the stress

A number of dimensions of stress remain to be adequately examined. For example, are changes in eating greater or less for acute or chronic stressors? And does the stress associated with major life events necessarily produce similar effects to the stress associated with more minor life events? Work in other areas has suggested that perceived stress is more important than measures of life events in determining health outcomes (George 1989). Heatherton *et al.* (1992) suggest that stress must be ego-threatening to produce impacts on eating. Heatherton *et al.* (1998) showed that emotional distress led to increased eating in dieters but only when the distress was ego-threatening (i.e. implied negative feelings about the self). Other research suggests that stressors which require active coping may produce different effects from those which require more passive coping (Obrist 1981). Stressors that disrupt time schedules may be particularly important determinants of overeating. In addition, there are variables that can ameliorate the effects of stress on eating (e.g. coping strategies, minor uplifts). Finally, the intensity of stress might be important. The intensity of a stressor has been considered as a possible moderator of the effects of stress on eating (Robbins and Fray 1980). For example, Stone and Brownell (1994) report that severity of stress was linked to the likelihood of eating less, such that eating less was particularly likely at high (severe) levels of stress. Conner *et al.* (1999) reported that although number of daily hassles was related to eating more snacks, the intensity of hassles did not have an impact on this relationship. Future research might usefully examine the impact of the nature of the stressor on eating behaviour and the role of coping strategies to mediate this relationship.

The nature of the eating behaviour

The major question that has been asked in research on stress and eating is whether stress increases, decreases or produces no change in eating behaviour. However, the impact of stress might also be upon the types of food selected. For example, Grunberg and Straub (1992) demonstrated that women were more likely to select foods high in calories (and fat) when under stress. Whether it is the high calorie content or the palatability of the food that is important has not been thoroughly investigated. Steptoe *et al.* (1998) reported that 'fast food' was eaten more frequently when respondents reported experiencing greater number of hassles. In addition, stress might produce impacts on the patterning of food intake. For example, Conner *et al.* (1999) showed effects of stress on the consumption of snack foods. Similar results were reported by Oliver and Wardle (1999) in a study of the perceived effects of stress on food choice. Snacking was generally perceived to increase under stress, regardless of gender or dieting status. In contrast, the consumption of foods usually taken as meals was reported to decrease under stress. Future research could usefully examine more specific predictions in relation to the impact of stress on eating (e.g. does stress particularly affect the consumption of palatable snack foods over other items in the diet?). Oliver *et al.* (2000) have undertaken focused work and shown stress to produce greater consumption of sweet high-fat foods and more energy-dense meals in emotional eaters.

The groups affected by stress

The existing research has examined a number of groups whose eating behaviour might be affected by stress. These include the obese, the restrained, women, emotional eaters and external eaters. The strongest evidence appears to be associated with the restrained, although the evidence here is almost exclusively in relation to young women. However, very few studies have examined these different groups simultaneously to determine which of the variables is the most powerful moderator of stress–eating relationships. Given the interrelationships of these variables, this is surprising. Future research could usefully assess which of the variables is crucial in influencing the relationship between stress and eating.

Mechanisms relating stress to eating

Although various mechanisms relating stress to eating have been suggested, very few have been systematically investigated. As we noted above, the general effect model of stress tends to suggest that stress produces biological changes. In contrast, the individual difference model of stress proposes that vulnerability to stress-induced eating results from a particular learning history. Future research could usefully formulate more specific hypotheses about the precise nature of these learning mechanisms.

Thus, in summary, future studies might usefully develop in several directions. First, we would recommend the use of larger-scale studies with diverse samples followed over prolonged periods, such as those employed by Stone and Brownell (1994). This would allow further examination of the various moderator variables within individuals in order to assess whether individuals show different patterns of responding and also whether these effects are similar across different populations. Second, examination of different types of stressors upon eating would seem to be warranted. For example, do uplifts (i.e. positive minor life events; Delongis *et al.* 1982) produce similar or the opposite effects upon eating to hassles? Finally, aspects of eating other than a simple measure of amount eaten might be examined. For example, does stress lead to greater consumption of food during meal times and as between-meal snacks? Does stress lead to the consumption of foods with particular characteristics, such as sweet foods (Grunberg and Straub 1992) or high fat foods (Michaud *et al.* 1990)? A further area of research that would be interesting to explore is the types of stressors that lead to eating, and whether particular types of stressors lead to eating only in particular groups of people. For example, Heatherton *et al.* (1992) showed that disinhibition of eating can be seen in ego-threatening situations, but not in physically threatening situations. Finally, hypotheses concerning the mechanisms underlying the relationship between stress and eating should be further investigated.

Summary

The research on stress and eating has produced a number of insights into the relationship between these two variables. The evidence for a general effect of stress on eating is modest and in general limited to animal studies. However, there does appear to be good evidence that stress leads to increased eating in restrained individuals. There is more limited evidence that being obese, being a woman or being an emotional or external eater are associated with stronger stress–eating relationships. Stress and disordered eating do appear to coexist frequently, although the relationship between the two remains to be clarified. Finally, much work remains to be conducted on the impact of the nature of the stressor, the types of eating behaviours affected, the populations afflicted and the explanatory mechanisms.

Suggested further reading

Ball, K. and Lee, C. (1999) Relationships between psychological stress, coping and disordered eating: A review, *Psychology and Health*, 14: 1007–35.
    This is an excellent review of the literature on the relationship of stress and coping to various aspects of disordered eating.
Conner, M., Fitter, M. and Fletcher, W. (1999) Stress and snacking: A diary study of daily hassles and between-meal snacking, *Psychology and Health*, 14, 51–63.
    One of the few studies to examine a number of the key moderators of the stress–eating relationship in a single study.
Greeno, C.G. and Wing, R.R. (1994) Stress-induced eating, *Psychological Bulletin*, 115, 444–64.
    An impressive review of the broad range of literature on the general effect and individual difference models of stress–eating relationships.

6

Food and social influence

General overview

Social influence can be defined in a number of ways. Broadly speaking, social influence refers to the perceived influence of one or more other persons. Social influence may be: direct or indirect; real, implied or imagined; conscious or subconscious. The preceding chapters have principally focused on the way in which individual psychology is influenced by the social world: for example, how attitudes are formed, how individuals use socially determined cognitions to change their weight and how responses to stress influence food intake. The emphasis of the present chapter is more exclusively on interpersonal influences on food intake: that is, the way in which people around us influence our food intake, either by their physical presence or by the ways in which we use food to communicate with them. Note that this maps on to the person-perception versus self-regulation distinction we made in Chapter 1. We start by examining indirect social pressure from the mere presence of others around us before considering more direct influences from the media. We then go on to consider the ways in which food is used both to communicate information about ourselves and to infer the traits of others from the food they buy or eat. The final section identifies a number of potential avenues for further work in this area.

Social facilitation

Norman Triplett is widely regarded as having conducted the first experiment in social psychology, published in the *American Journal of Psychology* in 1898 (but see Haines and Vaughan 1979 for an alternative view). Briefly, Triplett (1898) was interested in understanding why cyclists who rode alone were slower than cyclists who rode with others. His findings are often reported as showing that children in competition work faster than when working alone. Actually, the findings were less clear-cut than this, and the paper was largely ignored in the years that immediately followed. Eventually, the idea that the mere presence of others can profoundly influence the behaviour of individuals (**social facilitation**) was resurrected by Allport (1920), and has inspired a considerable amount of social psychological research.

The term *social facilitation* is somewhat misleading because the mere presence of others can also influence behaviour in an inhibitory manner. Zajonc (1965) argued that simple behaviours were facilitated by the presence of others, whereas more complex behaviours were inhibited. Briefly, Zajonc's (1965) drive theory proposes that the presence of others is arousing and that, in the presence of others, individuals typically revert to a *dominant response*. Thus, the performance of well rehearsed, simple or habitual behaviours is facilitated whereas more complex, less well learned behaviours are inhibited (for a review see Geen and Gange 1977). As a 'simple' behaviour, one might therefore expect eating to be facilitated by the mere presence of others. A number of animal researchers have demonstrated just such a phenomenon in a variety of species, from fish (e.g. Welty 1934) to gerbils (Forkman 1991).

In addition, social psychologists have been able to replicate this finding in human populations. A popular approach has been to pair participants with a confederate who consumes either a great deal of food or very little. For example, Nisbett and Storms (1974) found that when participants were paired with a low intake model, they ate 29 per cent less than when eating alone, but when they were paired with a high intake model they ate 25 per cent more than when eating alone. The implication is that the mere presence of others can exert powerful effects on eating behaviour. However, strictly speaking, these effects are not necessarily *mere exposure* effects and could be interpreted as the participants responding to an ambiguous situation purely by imitating the model (e.g. Zajonc *et al.* 1982) or by learning how to behave in that situation (e.g. Bandura 1997).

More recently, researchers have sought to control for these alternative explanations of the mere exposure effect by developing paradigms that do not include models. For example, Clendenen *et al.* (1994) compared ordinary people who ate either alone or with one or three other people. Comparable with the modelling studies, Clendenen *et al.* (1994) found that food consumption increased when participants dined with others, but that the number of people present did not seem to influence amount of food eaten. Thus, the mere presence of others was sufficient to increase consumption, although food intake did not increase further as companions were added. A second purpose of Clendenen *et al.*'s (1994) study was to examine the effects of individuals' relationships with their dining companions. Their findings indicated that participants eating with friends consumed more dessert than those eating with strangers. Clendenen *et al.* (1994) speculated that – given that desserts contain greater numbers of calories per volume – participants were motivated to project a good impression to strangers, but were more relaxed in the company of friends. In fact, a number of authors have investigated the mechanisms by which people with whom we are eating influence our own consumption, and we examine these throughout this chapter.

Thus, accumulated research suggests that eating in the presence of others increases the amount of food eaten. However, all the research described thus far was conducted in laboratories; in other words, artificial situations that allow for maximum control over extraneous variables, but possibly lacking in realism (see Chapter 1). Even when studies have attempted to mimic real life, such as Clendenen *et al.*'s (1994) 'Dinner and a Movie' study (where participants watched a short wildlife documentary prior to eating), the artificiality of the situations may have been the true influence on eating behaviour. For example, we know that people are motivated to bring order to their social world and often look to others to see how to behave in ambiguous situations, such as those often presented in the laboratory (e.g. Sherif 1936). Similarly, neither prior food intake nor regular eating patterns are consistently assessed before participants enter the laboratory and it is therefore possible that set meal patterns might be disrupted by laboratory experiments.

In response to the limitations associated with the experimental method, John de Castro has amassed a large body of evidence that examines the effects of social facilitation on eating behaviour in more naturalistic settings. Instead of asking individuals to snack or eat a single meal in a laboratory, de Castro and his group have assessed spontaneous eating in free-living human participants. The majority of these studies have involved asking participants to complete diaries of what they ate, with whom and for how long over periods of seven days or so. In general, de Castro's studies confirm the results of laboratory work. For example, de Castro (1997) examined results across 14 of his own studies (including more than 700 participants), and found that, on average, people ate 44 per cent more when in the presence of others than they did alone.

Given that de Castro's basic paradigm eschews the experimental method, it is more difficult to identify and control for a number of potential alternative explanations for these findings. For example, smaller meals (e.g. breakfast, snacks) are more likely to be eaten alone than are larger meals (e.g. evening meal), which are also more likely to be eaten in the presence of others. Evening meals in general are more likely to include alcohol and to be eaten in restaurants (both of which might increase overall calorific content), and meals eaten at the weekend might be larger than those eaten on weekdays. While it is clear that each of these factors is related to meal size, accumulated evidence shows that they do not account for the relationship between number of people and amount eaten (e.g. de Castro *et al.* 1990; de Castro 1991). Moreover, in an attempt to isolate a cause-and-effect relationship, Redd and de Castro (1992) instructed individuals to eat normally, eat alone or eat with friends for five days: more food was eaten by participants who ate with people.

Moreover, while controlling for such alternative explanations, de Castro's work provides insights that were previously obscured by the experimental method. For example, beyond the basic finding that the mere presence of people increases the amount consumed, de Castro and colleagues have shown that the number of people present correlates with the amount eaten. In contrast to experimental findings (e.g. Clendenen *et al.* 1994), de Castro and colleagues have found that the more people present, the more food is eaten. For example, de Castro and Brewer (1992: 124) found that: 'One other person present at the meal was associated with a 28 per cent increase in meal size while 41 per cent, 53 per cent, 53 per cent, 71 per cent, and 76 per cent increases were associated with two, three, four, five, and six or more people, respectively.' In other words, social facilitation of food intake appears to obey the law of diminishing returns: while eating with one or two other people greatly increases the amount of food eaten, once one is eating with four people, each additional person thereafter increases the amount of food consumed less and less. This basic pattern of findings holds when the effects are averaged across a number of studies (see de Castro 1997).

Interestingly, this pattern of diminishing social influence maps closely on to the 'psychosocial law' (principle 2) component of Latané's (1981) **social impact theory**. Originally, the social impact theory was designed to explain the phenomenon of *bystander apathy* – the finding that individuals are less likely to offer help when there are many others around them. By way of an example, Freeman *et al.* (1975) found that the larger the group of people dining together, the lower was the size of the tip left at the end of the meal. There are three principles underpinning social impact theory: social forces, the psychosocial law and multiplication versus division of impact. Of particular relevance to the present discussion is the psychosocial law (see Latané 1981 for a full description of social impact theory). The psychosocial law maps directly on to the findings of de Castro and Brewer (1992) and can perhaps best be summarized as the finding 'that the difference between 99 and 100 is less than the difference between 0 and 1' (Latané 1981: 344). Extending this law to de Castro's (1997) review, it seems that adding a fourth person increases the meal size considerably, but the effects of adding a fifth, sixth and seventh person produces smaller increments in the amount of food consumed.

Why do people eat more in the mere presence of others? A number of suggestions have been offered (e.g. alcohol consumption, meal type, time of day), most of which have been accounted for. However, there are two mechanisms that might provide further insight into the influence of social facilitation on eating: time and disinhibition. With respect to time, it has been found that people tend to spend longer eating when they are in larger groups. For example, Sommer and Steele (1997) surreptitiously observed people eating and found that those who ate in groups spent almost 15 minutes longer than those who were alone. Consistent with this, de Castro and Brewer (1992) found that not only did participants eat more in larger groups, but the meals also lasted longer. Crucially, de Castro and Brewer (1992) showed that people did not eat any more slowly when in larger groups and so the extra time was spent eating, thus leading to real increases in food intake. Therefore, given that the rate of consumption does not decrease, one possibility is that the mere presence of others increases meal size because of the extended duration of the meal.

The disinhibition hypothesis is based on the idea that people tend to exert cognitive control over their food intake, but that in the presence of others this control is relaxed. This may occur because people are distracted by the presence of others or perhaps because people feel more comfortable when eating in the presence of others. There is a growing body of evidence supporting the disinhibition hypothesis. For example, de Luca and Spigelman (1979) examined the effects of people eating with an obese confederate. While normal-weight participants ate the same amount regardless of the weight of the confederate, obese people consistently ate more when paired with an obese confederate than with a normal-weight confederate (de Luca and Spigelman 1979). Similarly, one study by de Castro (1994) found that family and friends produced greater levels of social facilitation than did co-workers, classmates or roommates (cf. Clendenen et al. 1994). Importantly, de Castro (1994) found that the effects were moderated by calmness: greater calm was associated with eating with friends/family; greater anxiety was associated with eating with co-workers. Thus, eating with friends and family may be relaxing and disinhibiting, whereas eating with co-workers and other acquaintances may elicit more cognitive control in an attempt to project a certain image. Social psychologists have been particularly interested in examining the ways in which eating behaviour is driven by impression management. We return to this issue later.

The work of de Castro and colleagues has been influential in providing an account of the influence of social facilitation on eating behaviour. However, his work focuses solely on indirect social influence, whereas most of us think about social influence in terms of direct effects. Indirect social influence can be regarded as those sorts of social influence that are not deliberately targeted at us, or do not deliberately set out to persuade us. Thus, the mere presence of others effect described above is clearly a form of social influence because the number of people you eat with affects the amount you eat, but the people you are eating with are not intentionally making you eat more. Direct social influence, on the other hand, is social influence that deliberately sets out to persuade us to do something. For example, government health campaigns might try to persuade us to eat a more healthy diet (see Chapter 3), or a child's parent may try to persuade her or him at least to *try* a novel food. Social psychologists regard this as a distinction between descriptive norms (our perception of what others around us are doing) and injunctive norms (the need to fit in with our social group in order to receive approval). This distinction was empirically tested by Conner et al. (1996), who found that both descriptive norms and injunctive norms were independently predictive of adolescents' intentions to diet. The following section examines arguably the most prominent source of direct social influence on eating behaviour: the mass media.

Effects of advertising

Advertising represents one of the more explicit ways in which social influences are brought to bear. The mass media are one of the most pervasive sources of advertising in our lives and encompass television, newspapers, magazines, billboards and radio. Each uses differing methods of advertising but they share the aim of encouraging us to buy the product being advertised or more of it. Food is one major consumable item upon which we all spend money and so it attracts a great deal of advertising. Advertisers capitalize on lifestyle changes to introduce new products, such as 'fast foods' and 'healthy' products. The motives of advertisers are threefold: to retain users of the product, to bring about switching to their brand and to induce new users to the advertised brand of a particular class of products (Schutz and Diaz-Knauf 1989).

Advertising performs another important role: that of providing information about product use; in other words, when, where and with whom we should be consuming particular food items. This might include information about what foods are healthy and which should be consumed in moderation. These aims are related to the perceived need of consumers to eat healthily and to lose weight. Hence, particular foods low in factors presumed to have negative effects on health (e.g. saturated fats, salt, calories) and high in factors presumed to have positive effects on health (e.g. calcium, fibre) have been consistently marketed over recent years to meet perceived consumer needs.

In Chapter 3, we discussed the way in which governments have tried to persuade people to eat healthily and it is interesting to note that advertisers use markedly different techniques to persuade people. In Chapter 3, we made a distinction between attitude change via central and peripheral routes (i.e. the elaboration likelihood model, Petty and Cacioppo 1986) and argued that persuasion could occur via either route. Broadly speaking, health promotion attempts have been targeted at the central route, whereas advertising is targeted at the peripheral route. Thus, while many health promotion campaigns seek to persuade people with strong arguments backed up with hard evidence (i.e. central route persuasion), advertisers tend to use peripheral-route techniques: branding, providing role models, mere exposure, message reinforcement, cued recall and so forth. Given that central-route persuasion should exert longer-lasting effects on attitudes, increase attitude–behaviour correspondence and be more resistant to counter-persuasion (Petty and Cacioppo 1986), why is there this disparity between advertising and health promotion?

There are two possible explanations for the apparent disparity between health promoters and advertisers: cost and audience characteristics. First, peripheral-route persuasion is simply more expensive than central-route persuasion. This is largely because central-route persuasion rests on the assumption that people will effectively 'persuade themselves' through their own cognitive responses, whereas the peripheral route works on the basis of repeated exposure and reinforcement. Repeated exposure and reinforcement is only possible with access to multiple media, and television in particular. Hence, advertisers focus their attention on television, whereas the medium of choice for health promotion seems to be the leaflet. Given that the vast majority of people in the West have access to at least one television, it is a potentially powerful form of influence and is certainly more powerful than written forms of communication (e.g. Chaiken and Eagly 1983). Although the peripheral route might be a less effective form of persuasion *per se*, access to multiple media seems to be a crucial persuasive asset.

To some extent, then, health promotion is targeted at the central route because of budgetary constraints. Paradoxically, the central route should also engender more effective attitude change, so why do advertisers not make greater use of it? The answer lies in the characteristics of the audience. On the one hand, health promoters are concerned with changing what might be deep-seated patterns of behaviour and where people have a greater personal involvement in the outcome. On the other hand, advertisers are trying to persuade people who are not personally involved to change their brand or to use a new product. Generally, it is easier to change the attitudes of people who are not personally involved than it is to change the attitudes of people who are personally involved.[1] For example, it would be relatively easy to persuade you to try a new type of chocolate bar with which you had no prior experience than it would be to persuade you to stop eating your favourite chocolate bar. Thus personal involvement affects the extent to which people are motivated to process a persuasive message – a key postulate of Petty and Cacioppo's (1986) elaboration likelihood model. Therefore, health promoters and advertisers use the central and peripheral routes respectively because of media and audience characteristics.

Much of the concern about the effects of advertising has focused on children, who are assumed to be more vulnerable to its effect. Children see a huge amount of advertising: it has been estimated that children in the USA are exposed to around 22,000 television advertisements per year (Lewis and Hill 1998). Moreover, it has been estimated that the majority of advertisements targeted at young children are for food products, and that up to 100 per cent of these are for foods that are high in fat, salt or sugar. For example, Lewis and Hill (1998) analysed 91.33 hours of television derived from a full week of children's programming. During the week of analysis, 828 advertisements were broadcast (about nine per hour). Of these, 49.4 per cent were for food products, the largest category by far. In fact, 'toys' was only the second largest category, and accounted for less than 10 per cent of all the advertisements. Thus, it is clear that child-targeted advertisements are typically for food. Moreover, Lewis and Hill (1998) identified five sub-categories within the larger 'food products' category. Their analyses revealed that 30.1 per cent of food product advertisements were for cereals, 29.8 per cent for snacks (both sweet and savoury), 21.2 per cent for 'convenience' foods (e.g. ready meals, sauces) and 5.9 per cent for fast food outlets (see Figure 6.1). That is, there was a clear bias towards unhealthy foods.

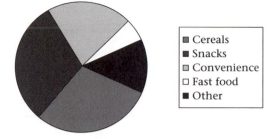

Figure 6.1 Type of food advertised as a proportion of all food advertising
Source: adapted from Lewis and Hill 1998.

Beyond this, Lewis and Hill (1998) examined the style and content of the different advertisements. They found that non-food products were more likely to emphasize value for money, while food products were more likely to be animated and humorous and to try to induce a positive shift in mood. Given that value for money is likely to be of greater concern to adults and perhaps older children, it seems as if the advertisements for food products were specifically targeted at younger children. It also appears that such advertisements are linked to a greater preference for the specific food items advertised. For example, Hitchings and Moynihan (1998) have found that there is a substantial correlation between the food advertisements that children recall and the foods they actually eat. It could therefore be argued that the majority of advertising that is aimed at children promotes unhealthy eating. For this very reason, the Swedish government has banned advertising targeted at children under the age of 12.

However, exposing children to advertisements for food items does not *guarantee* they will show a preference for these foods (e.g. Goldberg *et al.* 1978). In particular, while there is a clear relationship between advertising and consumption, it is almost impossible to deal with the cause–effect problem. In other words, it is almost impossible to tease apart whether advertising causes a change in behaviour or whether it merely reinforces what people are already doing. Indeed, when Lewis and Hill (1998: 212) tried to test experimentally the effects of food and non-food advertising on young children, they found what they described as 'weak and complex effects'. Many researchers would argue that the two processes work simultaneously (e.g. Schutz and Diaz-Knauf 1989). In some instances advertising does indeed merely reflect what people are doing in the market place – what they are buying, how frequently, what they think of the product etc. In other cases, advertising makes consumers aware of the products and leads to purchase. However, it is clear that the overall nutritional quality of foods promoted in advertisements targeted at children is poor and that there has been little discernible improvement since the 1970s (e.g. Gamble and Cotugna 1999).

In studies on adults, one focus of research attention has been on healthy eating (see also Chapter 3). Healthy eating is certainly something consumers are mostly keen to do. However, while many people report a willingness to eat healthily there is less agreement over what constitutes healthy eating in the public's mind. For example, Povey *et al.* (1998) found that people of different ages, genders and educational attainment levels had different views as to what constituted a 'healthy diet'. Similarly, those who were already eating healthy diets perceived a 'healthy diet' differently from those currently not eating a healthy diet (Povey *et al.* 1998). The problem is linked to the fact that many of the messages about what does and does not constitute healthy eating have changed and even reversed in recent years. For example, the UK government used to recommend that citizens should 'go to work on an egg' before concerns about the rates of coronary heart disease led them to promote foodstuffs that were lower in cholesterol. Views on healthy eating certainly do have some influence upon individuals' choices of foods; there is a general tendency to select foods that are perceived to be more healthy. This has been utilized by advertisers as a means to increase market share under the guise of health promotion. Certain health foods are advertised through positive or negative emotional appeals. For example, high fibre cereals are advertised with a negative appeal, reporting the health risks associated with insufficient fibre consumption linked to the information that cereals can provide much of the daily requirement. However, the extent to which advertising has had a role to play in determining people's healthy food choices or is simply reflecting the desires of individuals to have more healthy foods is almost impossible to distinguish. What is clear is that the public's concern over the health implications of consuming particular diets has increased over recent years (Sheiham *et al.* 1987), but the precise origin of this change is not clear.

Moreover, for many people, the most important health implication of food consumption is weight, rather than coronary heart disease or any of the other focuses of government-targeted health interventions. During the past four decades the idea of feminine beauty in Western culture has changed; extreme thinness or even emaciation have become the ideal (e.g. Toro *et al.* 1988). Perhaps not surprisingly, dieting and other efforts to regulate body weight have reached epidemic proportions over the past three decades. This is reflected in the numerous articles relating to weight loss in popular magazines, which steadily increased in number through the latter part of the twentieth century. It is also clear that dieting is beginning at a very young age, with some studies reporting dieting in girls as young as nine (Hill *et al.* 1992). It appears that even young children have an awareness of body image. For example, seven-year-old obese children have been found to have lower body self-esteem than their normal-weight peers (Mendelson and White 1982).

The role of advertising has been twofold. First, the media in general promote particular body images for both sexes. In their selection of certain types of models and actors, the media provide an ideal that we are expected to aim for (see Chapter 4). Second, the food industry has responded to the dieting epidemic by producing numerous 'diet' products that are promoted through advertising. Thus, the media promote slimming diets as one way in which we can achieve such slim body shapes (Toro *et al.* 1988). This has proven to be a particular problem for women: not only is the message predominantly targeted at women but the idealized female image is slimmer than most women are able to achieve. In other words, the media encourage women to attempt to achieve a body shape that is unattainable by most women. The prevalence and value placed upon particular unrealistic body images leads to the popularity of dieting, despite limited evidence for its success (see Grogan 1999: Chapter 4).

Thus slimming diets have become popular because of the desire to achieve particular body images that are promoted in the media. However, as with most advertising effects it is not clear whether advertising is merely reflecting or is actively creating demand for particular body shapes and slimming diets. What is clear is that weight loss is dependent upon many factors and the utility of slimming diets to promote permanent weight loss is questionable (see Chapter 4).

One of the most important changes in eating habits in industrialized countries has been the increase in the consumption of fast food either in or away from the home. It is estimated that more than half of what North Americans eat comes from fast-food chains, and in 1991 North Americans spent $25,000 million on convenience foods. Fast food has become a major part of our diet. A number of factors, including advertising, have been influential in bringing about this change. For example, lifestyle changes brought about by the changing role of women from full-time housekeeper to working full- or part-time outside the home have had an important role to play (Schutz and Diaz-Knauf 1989). Similarly, the increasing numbers of single-parent families and those who live alone has decreased the time available for food preparation and for eating. There has been a corresponding increase in the desire for foods that can be quickly prepared in the home or quickly obtained outside the home. In addition to these contributing factors, the advertising of fast food has played an important role in its popularity (e.g. Lewis and Hill 1998).

A number of studies have examined the factors that determine who eats in fast food restaurants. For example, Axelson *et al.* (1983) examined the beliefs that distinguished those who frequently used fast food restaurants from those who used them infrequently. Differences were apparent in the beliefs about the taste and nutritional quality of the food, the price, the choice of foods, not having to cook and the location of the restaurant. Those who were more inclined to use fast food restaurants were more likely to believe the food was tasty, of good nutritional value, cheap and from a wide selection. These individuals also placed greater value on not having to cook, and thought the restaurant was conveniently located (Axelson *et al.* 1983).

The convenience of foods is merely one factor contributing to the increased use of fast food. However, convenience has taken on great importance in developed societies, largely because of the low value placed upon food preparation time. Given that the pressure on the time available for preparing and eating food is unlikely to decrease, it seems likely that the fast food culture is with us to stay. In such a culture it is likely that consumers are going to demand better tasting and more nutritious fast food in the future. The issue of the effect of fast food on health is as yet unresolved (Heald 1992).

Food consumption as communicative act

Thus far, we have considered a range of social influences on eating behaviour, from the subtle effects of social facilitation to the more direct effects of advertising. As such, we have regarded food as a **socially inert** object. By 'socially inert' we mean that our discussion of food in this chapter has centred on the way in which consumption can be influenced by social forces. To some extent, we could simply have replaced the word *food* with almost any other object or behaviour, from playing football to purchasing a car, because these social processes are general and not specific to food. We would argue that food should not be regarded as socially inert because it possesses a communicative function that is fairly unique in social psychology (but see Ennis and Zanna 2000 for a review of the communicative function of cars). As we shall see, food does indeed possess the power to communicate. In particular, social psychologists have shown that individuals readily make judgements of others depending on the food they are eating (or are believed to have eaten), and that we often choose foods to communicate something about our selves. Thus, the following sub-sections deal with the kinds of processes that are likely to account for the effects of social facilitation and advertising: the way in which we judge others and the way in which we manage our impressions of self in a social context.

Social judgement

In developing an understanding of the psychological processes that underpin social influences on food consumption, it is important to establish the status of food as a social object. In other words, it is important that food *matters* as a concept with which to judge other people; otherwise, phenomena such as social facilitation are unmediated through psychological processes. Consistent with its position as a constant in all human life, accumulated research suggests that people are willing to make quite extreme judgements about others on the basis of relatively little information. Most people make judgements of others on the basis of stereotypes, which in the early stages of interpersonal contact are likely to be based on outward appearance. Stereotypes are cognitive short-cuts used to make generalizations about groups of people and guide our attitudes and behaviour towards them. Social psychological research has shown that some of the most powerful stereotypes are attached to body shape/physique.

Researchers have grouped physique into three **somatotypes: endomorphs** are round and fat, **mesomorphs** are muscular and **ectomorphs** are thin and angular. Each somatotype is associated with particular defining character- istics. Endomorphs are perceived as having few friends, getting teased, being lazy, sickly, ugly, sloppy, sad, dirty and slow. Mesomorphs are typically described as being the least kind and intelligent but as having many friends and being healthy, brave and good looking. Ectomorphs tend to fall in the middle on many traits but are also rated as being the most fearful, intelligent and neat (see Ryckman *et al.* 1989). In general, people who are overweight are judged negatively on a range of important traits. This is perhaps unsurpris- ing, given the desire for thinness (Toro *et al.* 1988) that pervades our society, but there are a number of psychological mechanisms that underpin these judgements.

Weiner (1995) has shown that many types of prejudice (relating to unem- ployment, alcoholism, depression etc.) are underpinned by attributions of responsibility. Thus, if people are regarded as being responsible for their negative outcomes, they are subject to blame and stigmatization. In contrast, if people are judged as not being responsible, they are given sympathy and support. This basic pattern of findings has been linked to weight prejudice (anti-fat attitudes). For example, Crandall (1994) found that anti-fat attitudes were related to a number of other prejudicial beliefs. Thus, people who held anti-fat attitudes were more authoritarian in their outlook, believed in a 'just world' (i.e. that bad things happen to bad people) and were more likely to be racist (Crandall 1994). The implication is that, for people with anti-fat attitudes, people who are overweight are responsible for their weight and lack self-control or denial (e.g. Stein and Nemeroff 1995). Thus, overweight people 'deserve' to be punished by social exclusion, anger and blame. Worry- ingly, these effects seem to occur regardless of the relationship with the person. For example, Crandall (1995) discovered that parents were less likely to support their daughters through college financially if their daughters were overweight.

Not surprisingly, researchers have been keen to understand the develop- ment of such attitudes, and have extended such work to examine normal- weight individuals. This work has tended to marry the work on anti-fat attitudes with societal expectations placed on women in particular. One particular focus of research attention has been on judgements of the amount of food eaten by women and men. For example, Chaiken and Pliner (1987) provided participants with four different food diaries that were manipulated on two key dimensions: whether the diarist was female or male and whether the diarist ate large or small meals. Women and men were randomized to receive one of the four types of diary. The participants were asked to read the diary and then judge the diarist on a number of dimensions, the critical ones being: femininity, masculinity, concern with appearance and attractiveness.

Meal size did not affect the rating of male diarists, whereas female diarists were rated as being more feminine, less masculine, more attractive and more concerned about their appearance if they ate smaller meals. The implication is that eating smaller meals is somehow an appropriate behaviour for women, whereas men are not judged on the amount they eat.

In a related study, Basow and Kobrynowicz (1993) asked participants to view one of four videos of a woman eating: (a) a small feminine meal (salad); (b) a large feminine meal; (c) a small masculine meal (meatball sandwich); or (d) a large masculine meal. Analysis of social approval scores revealed that when eating a small feminine meal, the woman was accorded greater social approval than in any other condition. The implication is that both the size of the meal *and* the content of the meal are important in making social judgements. Thus, people readily make social judgements of others on the basis of food consumption, but what is it about food that elicits these reactions?

This question has been addressed by examining the moral overtones that are associated with food. For example, Stein and Nemeroff (1995) examined the moral overtones of food and found that people who ate 'good' food (i.e. healthy, non-fattening food) were judged to be more moral than those who ate 'bad' food (i.e. unhealthy, fattening food). Thus social judgements of people on the basis of food consumption are likely to be driven by the perceived moral implications of eating certain types of food. Interestingly, the effects reported by Stein and Nemeroff (1995) are principally explained by the Puritan ethic and the 'you are what you eat' principle. Briefly, the Puritan ethic, which 'holds that one should be industrious and deny pleasures and immediate gratification to the self' (Stein and Nemeroff 1995: 481), maps very closely on to the kinds of beliefs that underpin anti-fat attitudes (Crandall 1994, 1995). The idea is that by adhering to the Puritan ethic, you will (eventually) be rewarded for your self-discipline. By the same token, any loss of self-control should be punished, rather like Crandall's (1994) finding that anti-fat attitudes were related to the belief in a just world. Stein and Nemeroff's (1995) data demonstrated that the Puritan ethic partially explained the relationship between food type (i.e. good versus bad) and moral judgement.

The second explanation for Stein and Nemeroff's (1995) finding is the 'you are what you eat' principle. This principle rests on the notion that people somehow take on characteristics associated with the foods they eat. Nemeroff and Rozin (1989) have demonstrated this belief in US college students. The students were asked to rate the average male member of one of two (fictitious) tribes, one of which only ate boar, while the other tribe ate only turtle. Consistent with the belief that 'you are what you eat', boar-eaters were more likely to be rated as possessing boar-like qualities (e.g. heavy set), whereas turtle-eaters were more likely to possess turtle-like qualities (e.g. good swimmer). Extending these findings to Stein and Nemeroff's (1995) study, the implication is that the moral contents of the food were transmitted to the consumer. Hence, 'good-eaters' were rated as being good whereas 'bad-eaters' were rated as being bad (Stein and Nemeroff 1995). These studies therefore demonstrate that judgement of morality is closely associated with various types of food and go some way towards explaining why people are so readily judged on the basis of the food they eat.

Self-presentation

It is clear that we are likely to be judged on the basis of the food we eat (Stein and Nemeroff 1995), or on the basis of the food people think we eat (Crandall 1994). However, this is not to imply that we are passive in this process. Given that we know that foods possess powerful signals upon which we base social judgements, it would seem strange if we didn't sometimes use this information to modify the social signals we transmit to others. Support for this is provided by an article in the *Chicago Tribune*, which reported that 'A recent survey of 500 people across England for the supermarket chain Somerfield reveals that the vast majority (71 percent) believe that the contents of shopping carts send out powerful messages about the persons pushing them' (D. Lewis, cited in Mistiaen 1997: 9). Thus, even in a relatively bland social environment such as a supermarket chain, individuals are clearly conscious of the goods they are buying. In fact, there is a lot of social psychological research that has investigated the way in which people use their preferences and attitudes to communicate with others (e.g. Katz 1960).

At the most fundamental level, food is used to communicate something about status, and it has been suggested that all cultures discriminate between foods of high and low status (e.g. Gelfand 1971). Indeed, people are quick to judge the status of others on the basis of the foods or brands they choose. An early study by Mason Haire provides a useful example. Haire (1950) provided women with shopping lists purporting to come from homemakers. The lists were identical, except that in one condition instant coffee was included, while ground coffee was included in the other condition. The participants were then asked to 'write a brief description of her personality and character' (Haire 1950: 651). Analysis of the responses revealed that the instant coffee elicited negative judgements about the homemaker: 48 per cent described the woman as 'lazy' (versus 4 per cent), and 16 per cent (versus no one) described her as a bad wife! While more recent tests suggest that people are now less harsh on instant coffee purchasers (see Fram and Cibotti 1991), this does show that food choices can communicate status.

More recently, advertisers and social psychologists alike have discriminated between products that perform a **utilitarian function** and those that perform a **value-expressive function**. For example, Johar and Sirgy (1991: 23) define a utilitarian advertising appeal as 'a creative strategy that highlights the functional features of the product', whereas a value-expressive advertising appeal is designed to 'create an image of the generalized user of the advertised product'. In other words, advertisers can appeal to the practical aspects of any product or to how owning the product will make you look to others.

From a social psychological perspective, Shavitt and colleagues (e.g. Shavitt 1990; Shavitt *et al.* 1992) make a similar distinction between products that fulfil a utilitarian function and those that fulfil a social identity function. The utilitarian function simply reflects the extent to which a product fulfils its purpose: consistent with expectancy-value theory (see Chapter 2), people are motivated to maximize the rewards they derive from a product. In contrast, the social identity function reflects the extent to which a product communicates a value, identity or other information about the self. In expressing a social identity, the product is likely to be salient to others, to signify group membership and communicate more about the self. Thus, a tin of baked beans is likely to convey less social information than a punnet of sheeps' eyeballs. In other words, not all foods are likely to elicit social judgements or communicate information about the self, and it is likely to be anything unusual or salient about the food or the meal that you are eating that will provide others with information.

By way of an example, Shavitt and Fazio (1991) primed people to be oriented towards either a utilitarian function or a value-expressive function, and were then asked to express their attitudes and intentions with respect to one of two drinks: '7-Up' or 'Perrier'. These two drinks were chosen because 7-Up is more closely associated with taste (utilitarian function) than social image (value-expressive function), whereas Perrier is more closely associated with social image than taste. When the primed function matched the function associated with the drink, the attitude–intention correlation was 0.85 (Perrier) and 0.86 (7-Up). However, when the primed function was not matched the correlations were 0.36 (Perrier) and 0.44 (7-Up). Thus, advertising products in terms of the impression they will convey is particularly persuasive, but it is important to identify which products are regarded as utilitarian and which are value-expressive. As far as we are aware, there have been no other attempts to look at specific foodstuffs in this manner, although it does seem as if the way in which one eats food and the amount that one eats are regarded as socially communicative.

The way in which one eats food can be used to communicate interpersonal relationships. For example, Miller *et al.* (1998) argue that the social sharing of food represents another form of communication. In particular, they identify three different types: food sharing, social feeding and food consubstantiation (i.e. where another individual has been in physical contact with the food). They hypothesize that sharing food suggests moderate intimacy that deepens with social feeding and even more so with food consubstantiation.[2] This hypothesis was supported in a questionnaire and video observation study. It was found that food sharing was indicative of a friendly social relationship. Social feeding usually indicates a stronger – probably romantic – relationship; additional consubstantiation increased reported intimacy and closeness of the personal relationship.

Earlier in the chapter, we described a study carried out by Chaiken and Pliner (1987) that showed that women (but not men) tended to be judged on the amount of food they eat. On the one hand, this is an elegant demonstration of the moral overtones of food and the effect of cultural ideals of femininity on social judgements. On the other hand, it also suggests that women (in particular) might use their food intake to communicate aspects of the self. Mori *et al.* (1987) extended the work of Chaiken and Pliner (1987) by manipulating the extent to which women were able to express their femininity. In their first study, Mori *et al.* (1987) manipulated the gender and desirability of participants' eating companions. Consistent with their hypotheses, women ate significantly fewer snacks in the presence of a desirable man than did women who were with undesirable males (or females). In contrast, men generally ate less in the presence of women, regardless of whether or not they were desirable. The implication is that men are less likely than women to use food in impression management.

Mori *et al.*'s (1987) second study adopted a slightly different approach by manipulating feedback on a masculinity test. It was hypothesized that women who were informed they possessed masculine traits would regard this as a threat to their femininity and would seek to redress this balance by eating less. In addition, Mori *et al.* (1987) manipulated whether or not the person with whom the participant was eating was aware of the feedback. Consistent with their hypotheses, women ate less when told they possessed masculine traits, but ate less still if the person they were eating with was aware of the feedback. The implication is that women's eating behaviour is modified by concerns about the way in which they present themselves, particularly in situations that highlight their femininity. These data suggest that cultural ideals can exert a powerful influence over dietary intake.

Pliner and Chaiken (1990: Experiment 2) further investigated the motives underlying such behaviour and confirmed that social desirability exerted a strong influence on amount consumed when eating with someone else. Interestingly, they found that this effect occurred regardless of whether the participant was male or female. For females, the need to look feminine exerted a powerful influence on eating behaviour. In contrast, masculinity was not an important determinant of male consumption. However, men tended to eat more when partnered with other men, which seemed to be motivated by competition (no such effect was found for female companions). Therefore, social desirability influences the eating behaviour of both men and women, although there are different motives underpinning the eating behaviour of women.

A related question concerns the extent to which these cultural ideals are internalized. The presence of other people in a laboratory, with appropriate cues to signal attractiveness, is the perfect arena for demonstrating the effects of femininity and masculinity on food intake. But what happens when people eat alone? As we have already argued in Chapter 4, eating disorders are characterized by secrecy and deception, so how might cultural norms influence people when alone? A study by Roth *et al.* (2001) provides some insight into this question. As we have already seen, social norms can override hunger and satiety as a mechanism for when people do and do not eat (Chapter 2). Roth *et al.* (2001) argue that people adhere to 'appropriate' norms for eating, specifically a matching norm and a norm for minimal eating. The **matching norm** is the kind of mere presence effect demonstrated by de Castro and colleagues: people tend to match their eating to others around them. In situations where it is important to make a good impression, the **norm for minimal eating** dictates that one should eat minimally. It is interesting to note that minimal eating might innoculate one against accusations of lack of self-control (Stein and Nemeroff 1995).

Based on this reasoning, Roth *et al.* (2001) asked participants to eat biscuits either alone or while being observed. They also told the participants that previously people had (a) eaten a lot or (b) eaten a little, or (c) they did not tell them anything. This manipulation was designed to provide them with some normative information. When unobserved, participants were influenced by the norms and ate more when told that other people had eaten a lot of biscuits. This suggests that the matching norm influences eating behaviour in the absence of a social influence source and implies that perhaps cultural ideals can be overpowered by norms related to particular situations. However, irrespective of the type of normative information they were given, people who were observed ate minimally, suggesting that the presence of others can trigger the norm for minimal eating, which is actually more powerful than the matching norm.

We began the chapter by considering the effect of the mere presence of others on eating behaviour and reviewed a body of work that demonstrates that people eat more in the presence of others (e.g. de Castro 1997). In contrast, the latter sections suggested that negative social judgements and a need to portray a positive self-image were likely to inhibit eating behaviour. At first glance, these findings seem contradictory, but unpacking them reveals that – as we have argued throughout the book – the social world exerts complex influences on eating behaviour.

In particular, it seems to be the *salience* of particular influences, such as femininity, that is important (Mori *et al.* 1987). Thus, in contrast with the work of Chaiken and Pliner, the studies conducted by de Castro and colleagues did not make factors such as desirability or sex role salient. Similarly, de Castro's studies focus on the naturalistic behaviour of people eating in groups. In the vast majority of eating situations, people will eat with people they know and are perhaps less susceptible to the kinds of pressures of cultural ideals. However, if the current preference for thin body shape continues, it may only be a matter of time before such factors are chronically salient in society. Having said that, de Castro's studies have tended not to analyse the gender of eating companions and so further work is required to resolve this issue. Similarly, Roth *et al.*'s findings need to be replicated in a more naturalistic setting.

Summary and conclusions

In this chapter, we have examined aspects of social influence on food intake. In doing so, we have examined social influence in the broadest possible way, referring not only to direct attempts to change our attitudes, as to advertising, but also to the presence and absence of other people, whether or not they are *trying* to change our behaviour. Generally speaking, we eat more when in the presence of others, unless we are somehow motivated to give a positive impression, in which case we tend to eat less than we would when alone. Quite when we are likely to be motivated to give a positive impression is not clear, although it seems to occur when we are most looking for social approval and when we are most likely to be influenced by injunctive norms. Similarly, the precise mechanisms through which norms affect us are not well known. Roth *et al.* (2001) have identified a matching norm and a norm for minimal eating, which seem to explain the way in which impression management works to influence food intake. Although these have only been tested in one study, they represent a promising area for future research.

To date, however, social judgement and self-presentation studies have typically only manipulated amount of food eaten (but see Basow and Kobrynowicz 1993). Given that some foods are more value-expressive than others, this seems like an important dimension that has yet to be manipulated. For example, what are the effects of eating large/small amounts of high- versus low-status foods? Presumably if 'you are what you eat', eating large amounts of high-status food should mean you are judged more positively. How this might fit with the norm for minimal eating is a matter for further research.

A parallel path for future research would be to examine further the mechanisms that explain these processes. Although we know about some of the kinds of norms that are likely to influence eating behaviour, tapping them directly is difficult, given that 'although people apparently conform and yield to influence because of concern with the opinions of others, it is not desirable to be recognized by others as being conforming or yielding' (Baumeister 1982: 8). Thus, self-presentational mechanisms can be used to disguise self-presentational mechanisms. It seems likely that the only way to gain further insights into these mechanisms would be to adopt some of the implicit measures of cognition, such as the implicit attitudes test (Greenwald *et al.* 1998), which seeks to measure cognition beyond conscious awareness. We return to this issue in Chapter 7.

Notes

1 Note that Johnson and Eagly (1989) distinguish between value-relevant involvement (i.e. expressing something about the self), outcome-relevant involvement (i.e. the person has a vested interest in the outcome) and impression-relevant involvement (i.e. the desire to express attitudes that are socially acceptable). Dietary change is

principally concerned with outcome-relevant involvement, which is most effectively changed with strong arguments (see Johnson and Eagly 1989).

2 Note that Miller *et al.*'s (1998) idea of consubstantiation maps on to the idea that 'you are what you eat' (Nemeroff and Rozin 1989); in other words, if you eat food that another individual has made physical contact with, the belief is that you will adopt some of their characteristics. The implication is that it is unacceptable to eat food that has been touched by someone who is a 'bad' person because it is 'contaminated'.

Suggested further reading

de Castro, J.M. (1997) Socio-cultural determinants of meal size and frequency, *British Journal of Nutrition*, 77, S39–S55.

Provides an overview of the work of de Castro and colleagues and addresses a number of possible alternative explanations for the 'social facilitation' effect.

Mori, D., Chaiken, S. and Pliner, P. (1987) 'Eating lightly' and the self-presentation of femininity, *Journal of Personality and Social Psychology*, 53, 693–702.

Classic paper that reports two experiments that manipulated the extent to which people presented themselves as feminine.

Pliner, P. and Chaiken, S. (1990) Eating, social motives, and self-presentation in women and men, *Journal of Experimental Social Psychology*, 26, 240–54.

Extends the Mori *et al.* (1987) paper with two experiments that examined the influence of social motives on behaviour.

7

Conclusions

This final chapter focuses on what we view as a number of interesting directions for future research in this area.

The social psychology of food

This book has attempted to illustrate the contribution of social psychological research to an understanding of food-related behaviours by focusing on research in a limited number of specific, but important, areas. In particular, we have examined food choice and social psychological models of the proximal determinants of food choices (Chapter 2). Similarly, we have examined the factors influencing changes in dietary choices (Chapter 3) and weight control (Chapter 4), and attempts to integrate these influences into stage models of behaviour change. We have also examined the role of social psychological variables that influence the relationship between stress and eating (Chapter 5). Finally, in Chapter 6 we examined the role of food in self-presentation. In this chapter we give more detailed consideration to several areas that offer interesting opportunities for further research on the social psychology of food. First, we examine social psychological research on more automatic influences upon our food choices. This contrasts with and complements the work on more controlled influences on food choice, such as the theory of planned behaviour presented in Chapter 2. Second, we give more detailed consideration to how models of controlled influences on food choice might usefully be further extended. The role of affective variables, attitude function and strength, and past behaviour are considered. Third, we give further space to the stage models of change that were presented in outline in Chapter 3. In particular we look at the role of volitional variables in such models and the implications for understanding maintenance of a behaviour.

Automatic influences on food choice

Russell Fazio (1986) has suggested that there are two distinct processes or modes by which attitudes can influence behaviours such as food choice. Where the individual is highly motivated and capable of thinking in a deliberate fashion, behaviour is thoughtfully planned and based on attitudes towards the behaviour (a deliberative process). The mechanism by which attitudes influence behaviour in this mode is thought to be described by models such as the TPB: implications of one's attitudes are reflected upon and, in conjunction with other information (about normative pressures and perceptions of control over the behaviour), an individual forms a behavioural plan (or intention) about how to behave. It is this plan or intention that guides behaviour. However, where motivation or opportunity for making deliberative decisions is missing, attitudes are held to impact upon behaviour through a more spontaneous process. Given the frequent nature of food choices, we might expect attitudes to influence many food choices in this more spontaneous manner.

Fazio (1986, 1990) employs the distinction between attitudes towards objects or targets and attitudes towards behaviours, and argues that it is the former that are important in determining behaviour via spontaneous processing. Thus Fazio is drawing upon the distinction between, for example, attitudes towards pasta and attitudes towards eating or buying pasta. According to the spontaneous processing model, an attitude towards an object/target may be automatically activated from memory following the presentation of relevant cues at the point of behaviour, with the likelihood of activation determined by the accessibility of the attitude (i.e. how quickly it can be recalled from memory). Attitude accessibility is, in turn, a function of the strength of the relationship between the attitude object and its evaluation in memory. Once activated, the attitude shapes the perception of the situation and produces attitude-congruent behaviour. Thus, if an attitude object activates a positive attitude this will lead the individual to attend to and notice the positive qualities of the attitude object (selective perception), which will shape the individual's definition of the event, and approach behaviours will follow. So, for example, if an individual has a particularly positive attitude towards salad, he or she will be inclined to notice the positive aspects of salad (e.g. healthiness, freshness) and ignore its negative aspects (e.g. lack of calories, not filling), and thus be more likely to choose salad over other available food choices.

Using response latency as a measure of attitude accessibility, it has been shown that quickly recalled attitudes correlate more strongly with behaviour than more slowly recalled attitudes (Fazio and Williams 1986; Fazio *et al.* 1989). A **meta-analysis** of attitude–behaviour relationships by Kraus (1995) reported that increased accessibility was associated with greater attitude–behaviour consistency. Research has also shown that variables likely to increase attitude accessibility (e.g. direct experience, repeated attitude expression) also improve attitude–behaviour correspondence (Powell and Fazio 1984; Houston and Fazio 1989). In relation to work with food these issues have been relatively rarely assessed to date. Studies have not examined the impact of response latency for attitudes towards foods and the vast majority of studies in this area work with foods and drinks that are not novel. However, Arvola *et al.* (1999) do report some relevant data. They examined the relationship between attitude and intention for two novel and two familiar cheeses. The attitude–intention-to-consume correlation was significantly stronger for the familiar cheeses (mean $r = 0.72$) than for the novel cheeses (mean $r = 0.52$). This would support findings from other areas that experience with an attitude object makes attitude a stronger predictor of behaviour in relation to that attitude object.

Thus, Fazio's work on the spontaneous impact of attitudes on behaviour can be seen as a useful complement to descriptions of the deliberative manner in which attitudes impact on behaviour, such as the TPB (see Eagly and Chaiken 1993: 206). A dual process model of attitude–behaviour relationships might provide a means of understanding this relationship. Where motivation and opportunity permit, attitude towards behaviour may well influence behaviour via intentions, as the TPB describes. When either motivation or opportunity is lacking the attitude towards the object might impact upon behaviour in a more spontaneous manner (Sanbonmatsu and Fazio 1990; Schuette and Fazio 1995). Fazio's (1990) MODE model (Motivation and Opportunities DEtermine attitude–behaviour relationships) might provide a useful basis for a more comprehensive understanding of the multiple processes by which attitudes can influence behaviour. For example, such a dual process model might help to explain how frequently repeated behaviours such as food choices gradually switch from being influenced by attitudes via a deliberative process to a more automatic or habitual process (Aarts *et al.* 1998).

Related to these automatic processes by which attitudes influence behaviour is recent work examining implicit attitudes as a complement to explicit attitudes (Wilson *et al.* 2000). Explicit attitudes are ones that the individual can consciously retrieve and verbalize. Such attitudes may be particularly relevant to important decisions. In contrast, implicit attitudes cannot be consciously retrieved, although the individual may be aware of them. They may be based upon previous experiences with the attitude object. The nature of the relationship between implicit and explicit attitudes is unclear. Implicit attitudes are assessed by methods such as the implicit attitude test (IAT; Greenwald *et al.* 1998). The IAT measures the response latency (time taken to respond) to pairs of items that are evaluatively congruent or incongruent. It is assumed that response times will be shorter when the pairs of items are evaluatively congruent than when they are incongruent. The strength of the implicit attitude is based on the average difference in response times for evaluatively congruent versus incongruent pairs. For example, implicit attitudes towards vegetarian meals would be assessed by presenting various examples of vegetarian and non-vegetarian meals along with evaluative terms such as good and bad. An individual with a strong implicit positive attitude towards vegetarian meals should be considerably quicker at judging pairs where vegetarian meals are matched with good and non-vegetarian meals are matched with bad than the reverse pattern. In contrast, an individual with a strong implicit negative attitude towards vegetarian meals should respond more quickly to the vegetarian/bad and non-vegetarian/good pairings than the reverse. An individual without a strong attitude towards vegetarian meals should not show differences in response times to these different pairings. Currently the majority of the work on implicit attitudes has been upon racial attitudes. Nevertheless, attitudes towards foods may be an important area for the application of these measures. This may be particularly the case where individuals have a disparity in their explicit and implicit attitude towards a food (i.e. a form of attitudinal ambivalence).

In summary, examination of the automatic processes by which attitudes influence food choice provides a promising avenue of research. In addition, cognitive factors other than attitudes might automatically influence behaviour (Bargh 1990). These factors might also be interesting in relation to various food-related behaviours.

Extending social psychological models of food choice

The theory of planned behaviour is probably the most widely applied deliberative model of attitude–behaviour relationships. As we noted in Chapter 2, the TPB has been used with some degree of success to predict a variety of food-related behaviours (Sparks 1994; Conner and Sparks 1996). The TPB details the determinants of an individual's decision to enact a particular behaviour, such as the choice of a particular food. In Chapter 2 we noted a number of extensions to the TPB (see Conner and Armitage 1998 for a more general review of extensions to the TPB). In this section we develop a number of interesting ideas for extending such deliberative models that may be particularly relevant to food choice. In particular, we look at the role of affect in food choices, the functions and strength of attitudes and their impact on food choices, and the role of past behaviour or habit in food choices and factors that might weaken the impact of past behaviour on future behaviour.

Affect and food choice

A common criticism of deliberative models such as the TPB is the failure to give adequate attention to the role of affective influences on behaviour (Conner and Armitage 1998). Such affective reactions to the performance or non-performance of a behaviour may be important determinants of intentions and behaviours (Triandis 1977; van der Pligt and de Vries 1998), especially for behaviours such as food choice, which are affectively laden. Some researchers looking at attitude–behaviour relationships for food choices have equated attitude with affect or liking (e.g. Tuorila 1990). However, more recent research supports more sophisticated views of the influence of affective factors on behaviour.

Much research in this area has focused on the influence of anticipated regret (Parker *et al.* 1995; Richard *et al.* 1995, 1998). It is argued that if an individual anticipates feeling regret after performing a behaviour then he or she will be unlikely to perform the behaviour. In particular, it has been argued that such reactions will drive behaviour when they are salient, or when they have been made salient. For example, Richard *et al.* (1996) reported that anticipated affective reactions were significant predictors of behavioural expectancy, after taking account of attitudes, subjective norms and PBC, for eating junk foods, using soft drugs and alcohol use, but not for studying. The effects of anticipated affective reactions have been confirmed in other studies of consumer behaviours (Simonson 1992).

Manstead and Parker (1995) make the useful distinction between affective reactions experienced after the behaviour and during the behaviour. This temporal dimension to affective influences may be particularly relevant to furthering our understanding of food choices. For example, one might find a slice of chocolate cake appealing because one anticipates the positive affect associated with the taste during eating the cake. However, one might also anticipate negative affect after eating the cake as one worries about the implications for the wasteline. We believe that the development and testing of these ideas might provide useful insights into the role of affect in food choices.

Attitude function and strength

In studies of the role of attitudes in food choices the function that the attitudes serve and the strength of the attitudes are concepts that have been relatively neglected. Attitudes are assumed to serve one of a number of functions or needs for an individual. Katz (1960) and Shavitt (1990) have noted four major functions that attitudes serve. The knowledge function presumes that attitudes can help to organize and simplify people's experiences. In the adjustment or utilitarian function, attitudes help individuals to maximize rewards and minimize punishments in their environments. Under the ego-defensive function, attitudes enable individuals to protect themselves from unpleasant realities. Finally, with the value-expressive function, attitudes allow individuals to express their personal values and self-concept. Relatively few studies have examined the impact of attitude function on the way attitudes relate to behaviour (but see Shavitt and Fazio 1991: Chapter 6). Work by Wilson and colleagues (1989) has demonstrated that thinking about why one holds an attitude can either increase or decrease the attitude–behaviour relationship (i.e. thinking about one's attitude seems to cue cognitive influences on one's attitude; if cognitive factors are also particularly accessible at the time of performing the behaviour there should be an elevation in the attitude–behaviour relationship; if affective factors are particularly accessible at the time of performing the behaviour there should be a weakening of the attitude–behaviour relationship). Clearly such research has important implications for the way in which attitudes are assessed and the likely implications for the actual impact of attitudes on behaviour. Further work on various attitude functions in relation to attitude–behaviour relationships for food choices is warranted.

Measures of the strength of an attitude appear to moderate the relationship between attitudes and behaviour (i.e. strong attitudes tend to show a closer correspondence with behaviour than do weak attitudes). This is probably because strong attitudes are more easily retrieved from memory when the individual is faced with the attitude object (Fazio 1986). Several measures of attitude strength have been reported in the literature (certainty, response latency etc.). However, very few studies have examined the impact of attitude strength in relation to food choices. This is a serious weakness in the present literature, which is commented on by Olsen (1999) and Lozano *et al.* (1999). The one exception appears to be in relation to the construct of attitudinal ambivalence. Some interpretations of attitudinal ambivalence draw upon a theoretical distinction between a traditional view of attitudes as evaluations stored in memory and a view of attitudes as constructions. This latter view suggests that attitudes are not stored in memory but are constructed when required (see Wilson and Hodges 1992; Conner and Sparks 2001). It is suggested that it is beliefs about the attitude object/behaviour that are stored in memory. These are selectively recalled when the individual is faced with a need to use their attitude to make a decision. What is interesting about this approach is that it focuses attention on the factors in the situation that promote the recall of different information. For attitude objects with which the individual has plenty of experience, the overall evaluation of the object may be the most easily retrieved piece of information. In contrast, for new attitude objects, the overall evaluation will not be relevant and other information will be used to judge the attitude object. In relation to ambivalence, it is suggested that to the extent that the pieces of information retrieved are evaluatively consistent, ambivalence will be lower and the attitude will be strong. In contrast, when the retrieved information is evaluatively inconsistent, ambivalence will be high and the attitude will be weak.

Several studies with food behaviours have demonstrated that weaker attitudes, as evidenced by increased levels of ambivalence, are poorer predictors of behaviour. For example, Sparks *et al.* (2001) report a significant moderating effect of attitudinal ambivalence on attitude–intention relationships such that higher levels of ambivalence are associated with weaker relationships for chocolate and meat consumption. Armitage and Conner (2000a: Study 1) used a prospective design and showed the same direction of effect on attitude–intention and attitude–behaviour relationships for consuming a low-fat diet.

Attitude strength measures deserve further attention in this area as potential moderators of attitude–intention–behaviour relationships. In particular, attitude certainty, attitude stability, attitude accessibility and the consistency between cognitive and affective elements of attitudes remain underresearched in the food domain.

Past behaviour and habit

The influence of past behaviour on current behaviour is an issue that has attracted considerable attention in this area (see Eagly and Chaiken 1993: 178–82 for a review). Because of the frequent nature of most food choices it might be expected that past behaviour is a particularly strong influence on future food choices. It is argued that many behaviours are determined by one's past behaviour rather than cognitions such as those described in the TPB (Sutton 1994). The argument is based on the results of a number of studies showing past behaviour to be the best predictor of future behaviour. For example, Mullen et al. (1987) used the theory of reasoned action (see Chapter 2) to examine changes in the consumption of sweet and fried foods, smoking and exercise over an eight-month period. For each behaviour, initial behaviour was the strongest predictor of later behaviour. Conner and Armitage (1998) reviewed a series of studies examining the role of past behaviour in the TPB. Across 12 tests of the TPB, after taking account of attitude, subjective norms and PBC, past behaviour was found to explain a further 7.2 per cent of the variance in intentions. Similarly, across seven tests, past behaviour was found to explain 13.0 per cent of variance in behaviour after taking account of intentions and PBC.

Ouellette and Wood (1998) provide a theoretical basis for considering when behaviours will be primarily determined by past behaviour and when they will be determined by intentions to act. They argue that for well practised (frequently performed) behaviours in constant contexts, past behaviour will guide behaviour because the processes that initiate and control performance become automatic ('habitually controlled' behaviours). On the other hand, for behaviours that are not well learned (infrequently performed) or are performed in unstable or difficult contexts, the impact of past behaviour on behaviour is assumed to be mediated by intentions ('consciously controlled' behaviours). Ouellette and Wood (1998) review a number of studies supporting this effect. At face value this research would suggest that the vast majority of food choices would tend to be habitually controlled because they tend to be well practised and occur in constant contexts. However, some recent research with food choices has challenged this view.

Conner et al. (2000: Study 2) looked at the predictors of eating a low-fat diet over a three-month period using the TPB. As predicted by Ouellette and Wood (1998), past behaviour was the strongest predictor of behaviour. However, the impact of past behaviour and intentions was moderated by the strength of the intentions and perceptions of control (PBC). When PBC was strong (as indicated by being stable over time), past behaviour was not significantly related to behaviour, and PBC was a strong predictor. Similarly, when intentions were strong (showed temporal stability), they were considerably stronger predictors of behaviour than when they were weak. Conner *et al.* (2002) show similar effects for eating a healthy diet over a six-year period. When intentions to eat a healthy diet were strong (stable over time), they were particularly strong predictors of behaviour, while past behaviour was not a predictor of behaviour. Together these studies demonstrate that even for frequently performed eating behaviours, which presumably occurred in relatively constant contexts, when cognitions are strong they can overwhelm the effects of past behaviour. Further research examining factors that moderate the impact of past behaviour on future behaviour in the food area could provide important insights into the factors that determine successful dietary change.

Aarts *et al.* (1998) provide evidence to suggest a mechanism by which past behaviour or habit determines behaviour. Where behaviour is habitual for an individual, he or she appears to be more likely to use simplified decision rules (i.e. enact the same behaviour as enacted in past). For example, Verplanken *et al.* (1997) found that those who had frequently performed a behaviour previously (using a particular mode of transport in this case), when given the opportunity searched for less information about which travel mode to use and were more likely to focus on information about the habitual choice than alternative choices, compared to those who less frequently performed the behaviour. It may be that past behaviour acts as a source of information. Aarts *et al.* (1998) argue that habitual behaviours become capable of being automatically activated by features of the situation and context in which the behaviour occurs (see Bargh 1990; Bargh and Barndollar 1996).

In summary, future research might usefully examine the factors that cause habitual behaviours to come under the influence of controlled processes such as intentions. As we noted above, the strength of cognitive variables, as indicated by their temporal stability, may be one factor that brings habitual behaviours under the influence of controlled processes.

Stage models of change in relation to dietary change

As we noted in the previous section, models such as the TPB can be characterized as deliberative models and are primarily concerned with the influences on people's decisions to perform a behaviour. However, recent research has suggested that there may be qualitatively different stages in the initiation and maintenance of a change in behaviour (see Chapter 3). One of the first stage models was put forward by Prochaska and DiClemente (1984) in their transtheoretical model of change, briefly reviewed in Chapter 3. In its most recent form DiClemente *et al.* (1991) identify five stages of change: precontemplation, contemplation, preparation, action and maintenance. Individuals are seen to progress through each of the stages in order to achieve successful maintenance of a new behaviour. Taking the example of weight loss, a topic reviewed in Chapter 4, it is argued that in the precontemplation stage the individual is unaware that his or her weight constitutes a problem and therefore has no intention to try to change it. In the contemplation stage the individual starts to think about reducing his or her weight, but as yet is not committed to trying to change. It is in the preparation stage that the individual has an intention to change his or her weight and starts to make plans about how to achieve this change. The action stage is characterized by active attempts to reduce one's weight. After six months of successfully maintaining a new lower weight the individual moves into the maintenance stage, which is characterized by attempts to prevent relapse and to consolidate the new body weight.

Several other stage models have recently been developed including the Rubicon model (Heckhausen 1991), the health action process approach (Schwarzer 1992; Schwarzer and Fuchs 1996), the precaution-adoption process (Weinstein 1988; Weinstein and Sandman 1992) and goal setting theory (Bagozzi 1992, 1993; see Armitage and Conner 2000b for a review). Although these models raise a number of interesting questions about the process of behaviour change, as yet there is far from overwhelming evidence supporting any one of them. There are several important themes running through each of the stage models. First, they all emphasize a temporal perspective, such that there are different stages of behaviour change. While the models postulate different numbers of stages, they all follow the same basic pattern from a pre-contemplation stage through a motivation stage to the initiation and main-tenance of behaviour. The important point to make is that these models are dynamic in nature; people move from one stage to another over time. Second, these stage models imply that different factors are important at different stages (Sandman and Weinstein 1993). For example, in the earlier stages information may be processed about the costs and benefits of performing a behaviour, while in the later stages cognitions become more focused on the development of plans of action to initiate and support the maintenance of a behaviour. We see two areas (not given detailed attention earlier in the book) as being part-icularly interesting in relation to understanding dietary change: the role of volitional factors and understanding the maintenance of a behaviour change.

Volitional influences

Models such as the TPB can be seen to be primarily concerned with people's motivations to perform a behaviour or achieve a goal and, as such, can be considered to provide strong predictions of intentions. However, even strong intentions do not always lead to corresponding actions. Reviews of the rela-tionship between intentions and behaviours report a wide range of correla-tions but it is clear that many people who intend to perform a behaviour fail to do so.

Distinct from the motivation to achieve a desired goal, volitional variables refer to strategies or plans that might be employed in order to achieve a goal or perform a behaviour (see Perugini and Conner 2000). It has become com-mon to distinguish making a decision to carry out a behaviour (forming an intention) from implementing it (Beckman and Kuhl 1984; Kendzierski 1990; Ajzen 1996). The former is considered to be primarily a motivational process, while the latter is primarily a volitional process (Kuhl and Beckman 1985). Recent advances in the psychology of action control (Gollwitzer and Bargh 1996) have begun to elucidate the determinants of goal implementation. Various factors appear to influence effort, continued commitment to a behavioural goal and persistence in the face of obstacles. For example, individuals who develop a clear plan of how to achieve a distant goal (e.g. eat a healthy diet) are more likely subsequently to achieve the goal and maintain it in the face of obstacles or barriers (Fuhrman and Kuhl 1998) in the eating context. Other aspects of planning can determine the relationship between intentions and behaviour (e.g. Kendzierski 1990). Gollwitzer and Schall (1998), for example, suggest that planning: (a) serves to guide people's attention to various goal-related opportunities and means; (b) suppresses doubt about the goal's desirability or the probabilities for achieving the goal; (c) helps to mobilize effort in the face of difficulties; and (d) helps with resuming goal-directed behaviours if disruptions have occurred. Such volitional variables may be important in the achievement of various food-related goals (e.g. dietary change, weight control). We believe that further research with these variables could provide useful insights into the processes underlying dietary change. For example, Sparks *et al.* (1996), looking at the volitional variables important in promoting dietary change, identified planning as a factor individuals take very seriously as an aid to the implementation of a dietary change. Research on planning and other volitional factors could help us to develop effective intervention to promote dietary change.

Maintenance of behaviours

Another interesting issue raised by consideration of stage models is the maintenance of behaviours and the factors that promote maintenance (see Chapter 4). Several different stage models of behaviour change include a maintenance stage. However, the important factors promoting maintenance are not clearly elucidated in these models. We believe that research aimed at providing a better understanding of the factors promoting maintenance of a behaviour could be particularly valuable, not least because most of the health benefits associated with changes in our food choices are dependent on the changed behaviour being maintained for prolonged periods, if not indefinitely (Kumanyika *et al.* 2000). Several factors could be important in behavioural maintenance.

In Chapter 4 we noted that several variables might be important in influencing an individual's decision to maintain a behaviour such as eating a low-fat diet. These include feelings of self-efficacy or perceived control over the performance of the behaviour. Schwarzer (1992; Schwarzer and Fuchs 1996) provides one account of how self-efficacy might influence maintenance of a behaviour. He suggests that successful maintenance is dependent on the implementation of an action plan that includes a set of cognitive and behavioural skills that help people cope with behavioural lapses, and thus prevent complete relapse of the behaviour. Perceived social support from others in terms of informational and emotional support could also be important in maintaining a behaviour. In addition, a continued strong motivation to perform the behaviour is likely to be important. For example, Conner *et al.* (2002) demonstrate that having stable intentions produced healthy eating behaviours over periods as long as six years. Volitional variables may also be important. For example, Kuhl (1985) suggests a number of control strategies that enable individuals to overcome obstacles and persist with a behaviour. These include emotion control, motivation control and strategies for coping with failure.

Rothman (2000) has focused on the decision to maintain a behaviour (see Chapter 3). He suggests that the decisions to initiate and to maintain a behaviour are both based upon outcome expectancies. Rothman makes a distinction between initiation and maintenance, in that the former is an approach process, while the latter is an avoidance process. The decision to initiate a behaviour is based on a consideration of the potential benefits of the new pattern of behaviour compared to the current situation (i.e. outcome expectancies). Initiating a new behaviour thus depends on holding favourable expectancies regarding future outcomes. Rothman conceptualizes initiation as an approach-based self-regulatory system because it is seen as an attempt to reduce the discrepancy between a current state and a desired reference state. In contrast, the decision to maintain a behaviour is based on a consideration of whether the received outcomes associated with the new pattern of behaviour are sufficiently desirable to warrant continued action. Thus, maintenance decisions depend principally on perceived satisfaction with received outcomes. Maintenance is thus conceptualized as an avoidance-based self-regulatory system because it is seen as an attempt to maintain the discrepancy between a current state and an undesired reference state. Rothman (2000) further suggests that satisfaction will depend upon comparisons of received outcomes with expectations about what rewards a new pattern of behaviour will provide.

Future research could usefully examine whether these motivational and volitional factors can be integrated into a model of the determinants of maintaining a behaviour. If such a model can then be shown to provide good predictions of maintenance it might usefully form the basis of interventions to promote the maintenance of behaviours such as eating a high-fibre diet or avoiding high-fat foods.

Conclusion

Food is an important part of our lives and, we believe, an important focus of research attention. Social psychology has been concerned with how our thoughts, feelings and behaviours are influenced by others. Such social psychological variables are only one of a number of factors relevant to our interaction with food and so they need to be considered within this broader context. Nevertheless, these variables appear important because of their status as proximal determinants of behaviour that appear to mediate the impact of many other more basic influences. Research from a social psychological perspective has made important contributions to our understanding of our relationship with food in a number of areas. These include our choice of food, the processes involved in dietary change, food and weight control, food and stress, and the relationship between food and self-presentation. Nevertheless, many exciting issues in relation to food remain to be addressed. We believe that social psychological approaches can (in conjunction with other approaches) continue to make an important contribution to furthering our understanding of food-related behaviours.

Glossary

Action: the stage at which an individual has successfully performed a health behaviour, but has done so for only a limited period of time (usually less than six months).

Action-outcome expectancies: the extent to which one exerts agency over one's destiny.

Anorexia nervosa: an eating disorder characterized by the relentless pursuit of thinness through self-starvation.

Attitude: a psychological tendency to evaluate persons, physical objects, ideas or actions in a positive or negative manner.

Attitude object: a person, physical object, idea, group or action that can be evaluated in a positive or negative manner.

Attitude strength: an attitude dimension, theoretically unrelated to attitude extremity, that increases attitude–behaviour correspondence, increases the stability of attitudes, increases the resistance of attitudes to persuasion and guides subsequent thought.

Attitudinal ambivalence: bidimensional conceptualization of 'attitude' that states that attitudes may be simultaneously positive *and* negative.

Behavioural beliefs: beliefs about the attributes of an object (or the consequences of an act) multiplied by the evaluations of the attributes (or consequences of an act).

Behavioural intention: a summary of the motivation required to engage in a particular behaviour and a decision to pursue a goal or perform an action.

Behavioural processes: five strategies (counter-conditioning, helping relationships, reinforcement management, self-liberation and stimulus control) by which individuals prevent relapse to earlier stages of change.

Belief: a thought about the attributes of people, physical objects, ideas or actions or the relationship (e.g. associational, causal, inferential) between two attributes.

Bulimia nervosa: recurrent binge eating accompanied by a feeling of lack of control over eating followed by purging, and a persistent over-concern with body shape and weight.

Central route: attitude change that is the result of elaboration.

Cognitive responses: the idiosyncratic thoughts and reactions that an individual has in response to persuasive information.

Consciousness raising: an experiential process that involves obtaining new information about a particular health issue (e.g. by collecting information about levels of dietary fat).

Contemplation: the stage at which people are *thinking* about making a change in their behaviour.

Control beliefs: the perceived likelihood of facilitating/inhibiting factors occurring multiplied by the perceived power of those factors to facilitate/inhibit action.

Coping appraisal: an assessment of one's ability to manage a particular health threat which takes into account response cost, response efficacy and self-efficacy.

Counter-conditioning: a behavioural process by which the problem behaviour is replaced with alternative behaviours (e.g. choosing low-fat options).

Cues to action: stimuli (e.g. symptoms, health promotion) that prompt people to take remedial action with respect to their health.

Decisional balance: the process by which people weigh up pros and cons in order to decide how to act.

Downstream intervention: behaviour change attempts that are made on a small or medium scale and are usually targeted or tailored.

Dramatic relief: an experiential process by which one deals with the emotional experience of change, such as unhappiness associated with not eating cream cakes when one is on a low-fat diet.

Ectomorph: thin and angular somatotype that is usually rated as being the most fearful, intelligent and neat.

Elaboration: the psychological process of attitude change in which individuals thoughtfully consider the information presented, generate thoughts and feelings in response to that information and change their attitude as a function of these cognitive responses.

Elaboration likelihood model: a model of persuasion that posits a central and a peripheral route to persuasion.

Endomorph: round and fat somatotype, usually judged to have few friends, to be teased, lazy, sickly, ugly, sloppy, sad, dirty, and slow.

Environmental re-evaluation: an experiential process that involves the identification of social and physical influences on one's behaviour, e.g. by identifying situations that might lead to eating fatty foods.

Evaluation: a judgement of the value of something expressed (e.g. is it good or bad?).

Expectancy-value theory: representation of a person's attitude as the sum of the products of beliefs about the attributes of an object (or the consequences of an act) multiplied by the evaluations of the attributes (or consequences of an act).

Experiential processes: five strategies (consciousness raising, dramatic relief, environmental re-evaluation, self-re-evaluation and social liberation) by which people are held to move to subsequent stages of change.

Explanatory model: a model that identifies variables that cause behaviour.

Fear appeals: health promotion messages designed to arouse negative emotional reactions in people and thereby motivate them to act.

Food choice: the process of choosing foods for consumption.

Food rejection: food that is not eaten because it is distasteful, dangerous, inappropriate or disgusting.

Goal: mental representation of an object that a person wants to acquire, an outcome one desires to produce or an action one wishes to perform.

Habits: behaviours that are elicited automatically.

Health belief model: model that posits perceived susceptibility, perceived severity, perceived benefits, perceived barriers, health motivation and cues to action as determinants of health behaviour.

Health motivation: the extent to which people want to preserve their health.

Helping relationships: a behavioural process that taps social support and the way in which people use their relationships with others to help them change (e.g. by forming pacts with friends to avoid eating fast food).

Implementation intention: a plan to pursue a goal-directed behaviour: 'I intend to do X when situation Y is encountered.'

Innate preference: genetic predisposition to choose sweet or salty foods and to reject bitter or sour foods.

Maintenance: the stage at which an individual has successfully performed a particular health behaviour and has been doing so for six months or longer.

Matching law: animals seek to maximize their success in obtaining food.

Matching norm: adjusting one's own behaviour to complement that of those in the immediate social environment (e.g. eating similar amounts of food to those at the same table).

Mere exposure: the finding that simply being exposed to the same object on a number of occasions is sufficient to induce a positive evaluation.

Mesomorph: muscular somatotype described as being the least kind and intelligent but as having many friends and being healthy, brave and good looking.

Meta-analysis: quantitative integration of research findings to derive average effects sizes and identify moderator variables.

Midstream intervention: behaviour change attempts that are made on a large scale, such as at community, worksite or school-level.

Minimal intervention: behaviour change attempts that isolate key mechanisms for change and target those specifically.

Motivation to comply: felt need to acquiesce to the expectations of specific significant others.

Neophobia: 'fear of the new', which in terms of food choice means avoiding new, untried foods.

Norm for minimal eating: implicit social rule that one should consume only small amounts of food in public when it is important to make a good impression.

Normative beliefs: perceived social pressure from specified others whose opinions are valued to act (or not act) in a particular manner.

Obesity: body weight in excess of the healthy range (for gender and height) by 20 per cent or more.

Optimal foraging theory: theory that states animals make a trade-off between food intake and energy expenditure.

Perceived barriers: the perceived impediments to engaging in a particular health behaviour.

Perceived behavioural control: a person's belief as to the ease or difficulty of performing a particular behaviour.

Perceived benefits: the pros associated with performing a particular health behaviour.

Perceived need: perceptions of the need to change one's behaviour.

Perceived severity: perceived seriousness of a particular health outcome.

Perceived susceptibility: perceived likelihood of a negative health outcome occurring.

Perceived threat: combination of perceptions of severity and susceptibility.

Perceived vulnerability: perceived likelihood of a negative health outcome occurring.

Perception: a mental process that uses previous knowledge to compile and interpret stimuli that are registered by the senses.

Peripheral route: attitude change that is the result of non-thoughtful inferences and associations (e.g. through reinforcement, repeated exposure).

Persuasion: the extent to which an attitude changes.

Precontemplation: the stage at which an individual is not thinking about changing health behaviour.

Preparation: the stage at which an individual makes some small efforts to change behaviour.

Principle of correspondence: the principle states that attitudes will be most predictive of behaviour when the measures of attitude and behaviour are matched with respect to action, target, time and context.

Processes of change: five experiential and five behavioural strategies by which behaviour change is achieved.

Protection motivation: an index of the efforts people will make to preserve their own health.

Protection motivation theory: a model that assumes that motivation to act is a function of threat appraisal, coping appraisal and protection motivation.

Reinforcement management: a behavioural process that involves re-evaluating the way in which food is used as a reward or punishment.

Response cost: an assessment of the costs involved in following a particular healthful action (e.g. by giving up a liked negative health behaviour, or through painful procedure).

Response efficacy: a judgement of the effectiveness of the proposed cure or health action.

Satiety cascade: the physiological process by which people go from a state of hunger to non-hunger or satiety.

Self-efficacy: the confidence that one has in one's own ability to act.

Self-identity: the extent to which people ascribe enduring characteristics to themselves.

Self-liberation: a behavioural process that taps commitment to change.

Self-presentation: the organization of self and appearance to achieve interactional goals.

Self-re-evaluation: an experiential process that involves the examination of one's beliefs and attitudes about eating healthily (e.g. a low-fat diet can be tasty).

Situation-outcome expectancies: the extent to which one's behaviour is governed by external sources.

Social cognitive theory: a theory of behaviour change, which posits situational, outcome expectancies and self-efficacy expectancies as key determinants of social behaviour.

Social facilitation: the idea that the presence of others enhances one's performance.

Social impact theory: a theory that encapsulates the influence of others on the individual. As people (i.e. additional sources of influence) are added, the total influence increases in a linear fashion until a certain point, when the rate of increase in influence slows.

Social influence: the perception (real or imagined) that other people are directly or indirectly influencing one's thoughts, feelings and behaviour.

Socially inert: an attitude object that serves no communicative function.

Social judgement: the process by which we make inferences about the social world.

Social liberation: an experiential process that is concerned with changes in one's social identity such that it is possible to see one's self as (for example) a healthy eater.

Somatotype: a stereotype based on body shape.

Stages of change: five developmental stages (precontemplation, contemplation, preparation, action and maintenance) through which people pass in attempting to reach a particular health goal.

Stimulus control: a behavioural process that involves the monitoring of potential triggers to the negative health behaviour (e.g. avoiding fast food while passing an outlet).

Stress: an aversive state in which the well-being of the organism is threatened because demands of the environment exceed, or threaten to exceed, the available resources to cope.

Subjective norm: generally perceived social pressure from significant others to perform or not perform a particular behaviour.

Tailored intervention: a method of behaviour change that is specifically designed for the individual.

Targeted intervention: a method of behaviour change that is designed for a particular subgroup.

Theory of planned behaviour: a model of social behaviour that asserts that behaviour is a direct function of behavioural intentions to act and perceived behavioural control. Underpinning behavioural intentions are attitudes, subjective norms and perceived behavioural control, which in turn are determined by behavioural, normative and control beliefs, respectively.

Theory of reasoned action: a model of social behaviour that asserts that behaviour is a direct function of behavioural intentions to act. Underpinning behavioural intentions are attitudes and subjective norms, which in turn are determined by behavioural and normative beliefs, respectively.

Threat appraisal: a combined judgement of one's own vulnerability to – and the severity of – a particular negative health outcome.

Transtheoretical model of change: a model of health behaviour change that encompasses five stages of change – precontemplation, contemplation, preparation, action and maintenance – through which individuals pass in achieving a particular health goal. The model includes decisional balance and self-efficacy as mediators of change, as well as ten processes of change that are effective strategies for change.

Unrealistic optimism: a bias in risk perception that means people believe they are less at risk of negative outcomes, but more 'at risk' of positive outcomes than others who are like them.

Upstream intervention: behaviour change attempts that are made at governmental/policy level.

Utilitarian function: the holding of certain attitudes, the possession of certain artefacts or engagement in social behaviours to fulfil a practical purpose.

Value-expressive function: the holding of certain attitudes, the possession of certain artefacts or engagement in social behaviours to communicate information about the self.

Volition: the mental faculty of willing or trying to act. Volition is thought to be the mental event that produces bodily movements (i.e. action or behaviour).

Weight control: the outcome of the balance between energy consumed and expended.

References

Aarts, H., Verplanken, B. and van Knippenberg, A. (1998) Predicting behavior from actions in the past: repeated decision-making or a matter of habit, *Journal of Applied Social Psychology*, 28: 1355–74.

Ajzen, I. (1988) *Attitudes, Personality and Behavior*. Milton Keynes: Open University Press.

Ajzen, I. (1991) The theory of planned behavior, *Organizational Behavior and Human Decision Processes*, 50: 179–211.

Ajzen, I. (1996) The directive influence of attitudes on behavior, in P. Gollwitzer and J.A. Bargh (eds) *Psychology of Action*. New York: Guilford Press.

Ajzen, I. (1998) Models of human social behavior and their application to health psychology, *Psychology and Health*, 13: 735–9.

Ajzen, I. (2001) Nature and operation of attitudes, *Annual Review of Psychology*, 52: 27–58.

Ajzen, I. and Fishbein, M. (1977) Attitude–behavior relations: a theoretical analysis and review of empirical research, *Psychological Bulletin*, 84: 888–918.

Ajzen, I. and Fishbein, M. (1980) *Understanding Attitudes and Predicting Social Behavior*. Englewood Cliffs, NJ: Prentice Hall.

Ajzen, I. and Fishbein, M. (2000) Attitudes and the attitude–behavior relation: reasoned and automatic processes, *European Review of Social Psychology*, 11: 1–33.

Albarracin, D. and Wyer, R.S. Jr (2000) The cognitive impact of past behavior: Influences on beliefs, attitudes, and future behavioral decisions, *Journal of Personality and Social Psychology*, 79: 5–22.

Allport, F.H. (1920) The influence of the group upon association and thought, *Journal of Experimental Psychology*, 3: 159–82.

Allport, G.W. (1935) Attitudes, in C. Murchison (ed.) *Handbook of Social Psychology*. Worcester, MA: Clark University Press.

American Psychiatric Association (1994) *Diagnostic and Statistical Manual of Mental Disorders*, 4th edn. Washington, DC: APA.

Amerine, M.A., Pangborn, R.M. and Roessler, E.B. (1965) *Principles of Sensory Evaluation of Food*. New York: Academic Press.

Anderson, A.S., Cox, D.N., McKellar, S., *et al.* (1998) Take Five, a nutrition education intervention to increase fruit and vegetable intakes: impact on attitudes towards dietary change, *British Journal of Nutrition*, 80: 133–40.

Anderson, A.S. and Shepherd, R. (1989) Beliefs and attitudes toward 'healthier eating' among women attending maternity hospital, *Journal of Nutrition Education*, 21: 208–13.

Antelman, S.M., Szechtman, H., Chin, P. and Fisher, A.E. (1975) Tail pinch-induced eating, gnawing, and licking behavior in rats: dependence on the nigrostriatal dopamine system, *Brain Research*, 99: 319–37.

Armitage, C.J. and Arden, M.A. (2002) Exploring discontinuity patterns in the transtheoretical model: an application of the theory of planned behaviour, *British Journal of Health Psychology*, 7: 89–103.

Armitage, C.J. and Conner, M. (1999a) Distinguishing perceptions of control from self-efficacy: predicting consumption of a low-fat diet using the theory of planned behavior, *Journal of Applied Social Psychology*, 29: 72–90.

Armitage, C.J. and Conner, M. (1999b) Predictive validity of the theory of planned behaviour: the role of questionnaire format and social desirability, *Journal of Community and Applied Social Psychology*, 9: 261–72.

Armitage, C.J. and Conner, M. (2000a) The effects of ambivalence on attitude stability and pliability, prediction of behavior, and information processing, *Personality and Social Psychology Bulletin*, 26: 1432–43.

Armitage, C.J. and Conner, M. (2000b) Social cognition models and health behaviour: a structured review, *Psychology and Health*, 15: 173–89.

Armitage, C.J. and Conner, M. (2001a) Efficacy of a minimal intervention to reduce fat intake, *Social Science and Medicine*, 52: 1517–24.

Armitage, C.J. and Conner, M. (2001b) Efficacy of the theory of planned behaviour: a meta-analytic review, *British Journal of Social Psychology*, 40: 471–99.

Armitage, C.J. and Conner, M. (2002) Reducing fat intake: interventions based on the theory of planned behaviour, in D.R. Rutter and L. Quine (eds) *Changing Health Behaviour: Intervention and Research with Social Cognition Models*. Buckingham: Open University Press.

Armitage, C.J., Sheeran, P., Conner, M. and Arden, M.A. (2002) Stages of change versus changes of stage: predicting stage transitions in the transtheoretical model. Unpublished raw data, University of Sheffield.

Arvola, A., Lahteenmaki, L. and Tuorila, H. (1999) Predicting the intent to purchase unfamiliar and familiar cheeses: the effects of attitudes, expected liking and food neophobia, *Appetite*, 32: 113–26.

Assanand, S., Pinel, J.P.J. and Lehman, D.R. (1998) Personal theories of hunger and eating, *Journal of Applied Social Psychology*, 28: 998–1015.

Austoker, J. (1994) Diet and cancer, *British Medical Journal*, 308: 1610–14.

Axelson, M.L., Brinberg, D. and Durand, J.H. (1983) Eating at a fast-food restaurant: a social-psychological analysis, *Journal of Nutrition Education*, 15: 94–8.

Bagiella, E., Cairella, M., del Ben, M. and Godi, R. (1991) Changes in attitude toward food by obese patients treated with placebo and serotoninergic agents, *Current Therapeutic Research*, 50: 205–10.

Bagozzi, R.P. (1992) The self-regulation of attitudes, intentions and behaviour, *Social Psychology Quarterly*, 55: 178–204.

Bagozzi, R.P. (1993) On the neglect of volition in consumer research: a critique and proposal, *Psychology and Marketing*, 10: 215–37.

Bagozzi, R.P. and Edwards, E.A. (1998) Goal setting and goal pursuit in the regulation of body weight, *Psychology and Health*, 13: 593–621.

Bagozzi, R.P. and Edwards, E.A. (2000) Goal-striving and the implementation of goal intentions in the regulation of body weight, *Psychology and Health*, 15: 255–70.

Bagozzi, R.P. and Kimmel, S.K. (1995) A comparison of leading theories for the prediction of goal-directed behaviours, *British Journal of Social Psychology*, 34: 437–61.

Bagozzi, R.P. and Warshaw, P.R. (1990) Trying to consume, *Journal of Consumer Research*, 17: 127–41.

Ball, K. and Lee, C. (1999) Relationships between psychological stress, coping and disordered eating: a review, *Psychology and Health*, 14: 1007–35.

Bandura, A. (1982) Self-efficacy mechanism in human agency, *American Psychologist*, 37: 122–47.

Bandura, A. (1986) *Social Foundations of Thought and Action*. Englewood Cliffs, NJ: Prentice Hall.

Bandura, A. (1997) *Self-efficacy: The Exercise of Control*. New York: W.H. Freeman and Company.

Bandura, A. (2001) Social cognitive theory: an agentic perspective, *Annual Review of Psychology*, 52: 1–26.

Baranowski, T., Cullen, K.W. and Baranowski, J. (1999) Psychosocial correlates of dietary intake: advancing dietary intervention, *Annual Review of Nutrition*, 19: 17–40.

Bargh, J.A. (1990) Auto-motives: preconscious determinants of thought and behavior, in E.T. Higgins and R.M. Sorrentino (eds) *Handbook of Motivation and Cognition: Foundations of Social Behavior, Volume 2*. New York: Guilford Press.

Bargh, J.A. (1997) The automaticity of everyday life, in R.S. Wyer Jr (ed.) *Advances in Social Cognition*. Mahwah, NJ: Erlbaum.

Bargh, J.A. and Barndollar, K. (1996) Automaticity in action: the unconscious as repository of chronic goals and motives, in P. Gollwitzer and J.A. Bargh (eds) *Psychology of Action*. New York: Guilford Press.

Bargh, J.A., Chen, M. and Burrows, L. (1996) Automaticity of social behavior: direct effects of trait construct and stereotype activation on action, *Journal of Personality and Social Psychology*, 71: 230–44.

Baron, R.M. and Kenny, D.A. (1986) The moderator–mediator variable distinction in social psychological research: conceptual, strategic, and statistical considerations, *Journal of Personality and Social Psychology*, 51: 1173–82.

Basow, S.A. and Kobrynowicz, K. (1993) What is she eating? The effects of meal size on impressions of a female eater, *Sex Roles*, 23: 335–44.

Baumcom, D.H. and Aiken, P.A. (1981) Effects of depressed mood on eating among obese and nonobese dieting and nondieting persons, *Journal of Personality and Social Psychology*, 41: 577–85.

Baumeister, R.F. (1982) A self-presentational view of social phenomena, *Psychological Bulletin*, 91: 3–26.

Beardsworth, A. (1995) The management of food ambivalence: erosion or reconstruction?, in D. Maurer and J. Sobal (eds) *Eating Agendas: Food and Nutrition as Social Problems*. New York: De Gruyter.

Beauchamp, G.K. and Moran, M. (1984) Acceptance of sweet and salty tastes in 2–year-old children, *Appetite*, 5: 291–305.

Beckman, J. and Kuhl, J. (1984) Altering information to gain action control: functional aspects of human information-processing in decision making, *Journal of Research in Personality*, 18: 224–37.

Bellisle, F., Louis-Sylvestre, J., Linet, N., *et al.* (1990) Anxiety and food intake in men, *Psychosomatic Medicine*, 52: 452–7.

Beresford, S.A.A., Curry, S.J., Kristal, A.R., *et al.* (1997) A dietary intervention in primary care practice: the eating patterns study, *American Journal of Public Health*, 87: 610–16.

Bertino, M., Beauchamp, G.K. and Engleman, K. (1982) Long-term reduction in dietary sodium alters the taste of salt, *American Journal of Clinical Nutrition*, 36: 1134–44.

Birch, L.L. (1980) Effects of peer models' food choices and eating behaviors on preschoolers' food preferences, *Child Development*, 51: 489–96.

Birch, L.L. (1987) The acquisition of food acceptance patterns in children, in R. Boakes, D. Popplewell and M. Burton (eds) *Eating Habits*. Chichester: Wiley.

Birch, L.L. (1999) Development of food preferences, *Annual Review of Nutrition*, 19: 41–62.

Birch, L.L. and Marlin, D.W. (1982) I don't like it; I never tried it: effects of exposure to food on two-year-old children's food preferences, *Appetite*, 4: 353–60.

Birch, L.L., Marlin, D.W. and Rotter, J. (1984) Eating as the 'means' activity in contingency: effects on young children's food preference, *Child Development*, 55: 431–9.

Birch, L.L., Zimmerman, S. and Hind, H. (1980) The influence of social-affective context on preschool children's food preferences, *Child Development*, 51: 856–61.

Bjorntorp, P. (1987) Fat cell distribution and metabolism, in R.J. Wurtman and J.J. Wurtman (eds) *Human Obesity*. New York: New York Academy of Sciences.

Blair, A.J., Booth, D.A., Lewis, V.J. and Wainwright, C.J. (1989) The relative success of official and informal weight reduction techniques: retrospective correlational evidence, *Psychology and Health*, 3: 195–206.

Blair, A.J., Lewis, V.J. and Booth, D.A. (1990) Does emotional eating interfere with attempts at weight control in women?, *Appetite*, 15: 151–7.

Blaxter, M. (1990) *Health and Lifestyles*. London: Routledge.

Blundell, J.E. and Rogers, P.J. (1991) The satiating power of food, in *Encyclopedia of Human Biology*, Orlando: Academic Press, 6: 723–33.

Boeing, H., Jedrychowski, W., Wahrendorf, J., *et al.* (1991) Dietary risk factors in intestinal and diffuse types of stomach cancer: a multi-center case–control study in Poland, *Cancer Causes and Control*, 2: 227–33.

Boer, H. and Seydel, E.R. (1996) Protection motivation theory, in M. Conner and P. Norman (eds) *Predicting Health Behaviour*. Buckingham: Open University Press.

Booth, D.A. (1972) Postadsorptively induced suppression of appetite and the energostatic control of feeding, *Physiology and Behavior*, 9: 199–202.

Booth, D.A. (1985) Food-conditioned eating preferences and aversions with interoceptive elements: learned appetites and satieties, *Annals of the New York Academy of Science*, 443: 22–41.

Booth, D.A. and Conner, M.T. (1990) Characterisation and measurement of influences on food acceptability by analysis of choice differences: theory and practice, *Food Quality and Preference*, 2: 75–85.

Booth, D.A., Lewis, V.J. and Blair, A.J. (1989) Dietary restraint and binge eating: pseudo-quantitative anthropology for a medicalised problem habit, *Appetite*, 14: 116–19.

Booth, D.A. and Shepherd, R. (1988) Sensory influences on food acceptance: the neglected approach to nutrition promotion, *British Nutrition Foundation Nutrition Bulletin*, 13: 39–54.

Broughton, J.M. (1994) Declines in mammalian foraging efficiency during the Late Holocene, San Francisco Bay, California, *Journal of Anthropological Archaeology*, 13: 371–401.

Brown, L., Rosner, B., Willett, W.W. and Sacks, F.M. (1999) Cholesterol-lowering effects of dietary fiber: a meta-analysis, *American Journal of Clinical Nutrition*, 69: 30–42.

Brownell, K.D. and Rodin, J. (1994) The dieting maelstrom: Is it possible and advisable to lose weight?, *American Psychologist*, 49: 781–91.

Brownell, K.D. and Wadden, T.A. (1992) Etiology and treatment of obesity: understanding a serious, prevalent, and refactory disorder, *Journal of Consulting and Clinical Psychology*, 60: 505–17.

Bruch, H. (1973) *Eating Disorders: Obesity, Anorexia Nervosa and the Person Within*. New York: Basic Books.

Brug, J., Campbell, M. and van Assema, P. (1999) The application and impact of computer-generated personalized nutrition education: a review of the literature, *Patient Education and Counseling*, 36: 145–56.

Brunner, E., White, I., Thorogood, M., *et al.* (1997) Can dietary interventions change diet and cardiovascular risk factors? A meta-analysis of randomized controlled trials, *American Journal of Public Health*, 87: 1415–22.

Cade, J.E. and Margetts, B.M. (1988) Nutrient sources in the English diet: quantitative data from three English towns, *International Journal of Epidemiology*, 17: 844–8.

Campbell, M.K., de Vellis, B.M., Strecher, V.J., *et al.* (1994) Improving dietary behavior: the effectiveness of tailored messages in primary care settings, *American Journal of Public Health*, 84: 783–7.

Capaldi, E.D. (1996) *Why We Eat What We Eat: The Psychology of Eating*. Washington, DC: American Psychological Association.

Carver, C.S. and Scheier, M. (1990) Principles of self-regulation: action and emotion, in E.T. Higgins and R. Sorrentino (eds) *Handbook of Motivation and Cognition: Foundations of Social Behavior, Volume 2*. New York: Guilford Press.

Cash, T. (1990) The psychology of physical appearance: aesthetics, attributes, and images, in T. Cash and T. Pruzinsky (eds) *Body Images: Development, Deviance and Change*. New York: Guilford Press.

Chaiken, S. (1980) Heuristic versus systematic processing and the use of source versus message cues in persuasion, *Journal of Personality and Social Psychology*, 39: 752–66.

Chaiken, S. and Eagly, A.H. (1983) Communication modality as a determinant of persuasion: the role of communicator salience, *Journal of Personality and Social Psychology*, 45: 241–56.

Chaiken, S. and Pliner, P. (1987) Women, but not men are what they eat: the effect of meal size and gender on perceived femininity and masculinity, *Personality and Social Psychology Bulletin*, 13: 166–76.

Charles, N. and Kerr, M. (1986) Food for feminist thought, *Sociological Review*, 34: 537–72.

Charng, H.-W., Piliavin, J.A. and Callero, P. (1988) Role identity and reasoned action in the prediction of repeated behavior, *Social Psychology Quarterly*, 51: 303–17.

Cheng, K.K., Day, N.E., Duffy, S.W., *et al.* (1992) Pickled vegetables in the aetiology of oesophageal cancer in Hong Kong Chinese, *The Lancet*, 339: 1314–18.

Chesters, L. (1994) Women's talk: food, weight and body image, *Feminism and Psychology*, 4: 449–57.

Chew, F., Palmer, S. and Kim, S. (1998) Testing the influence of the health belief model and a television program on nutrition behavior, *Health Communication*, 10: 227–45.

Clendenen, V.I., Herman, C.P. and Polivy, J. (1994) Social facilitation of eating among friends and strangers, *Appetite*, 23: 1–13.

Cohen, S., Kamarck, T. and Mermelstein, R. (1983) A global measure of perceived stress, *Journal of Health and Social Behavior*, 24: 385–96.

Conner, M. (1991) Sweetness and food selection, in J.R. Piggott and S. Marie (eds) *A Handbook of Sweetness*. Glasgow: Blackie.

Conner, M. (2000) Meta-analysis of the attitude-behaviour relationship in food choice. Unpublished raw data, School of Psychology, University of Leeds.

Conner, M. and Abraham, C. (2001) Conscientiousness and the theory of planned behavior: towards a more complete model of the antecedents of intentions and behavior, *Personality and Social Psychology Bulletin*, 27: 1547–61.

Conner, M. and Armitage, C.J. (1998) Extending the theory of planned behavior: a review and avenues for further research, *Journal of Applied Social Psychology*, 28: 1429–64.

Conner, M.T. and Booth, D.A. (1988) Preferred sweetness of a lime drink and preference for sweet over non-sweet foods, related to sex and reported age and body-weight, *Appetite*, 10: 25–35.

Conner, M.T. and Booth, D.A. (1992) Combined measurement of food taste and consumer preference in the individual: reliability, precision and stability data, *Journal of Food Quality*, 15: 1–17.

Conner, M.T., Booth, D.A., Clifton, V.J. and Griffiths, R.P. (1988a) Individualised optimisation of liking of salt content of white bread, *Journal of Food Science*, 53: 549–54.

Conner, M., Fitter, M. and Fletcher, W. (1999) Stress and snacking: a diary study of daily hassles and between-meal snacking, *Psychology and Health*, 14: 51–63.

Conner, M.T., Haddon, A.V. and Booth, D.A. (1986) Very rapid, precise assessment of effects of constituent variation on product acceptability: consumer sweetness preferences in a lime drink, *Lebensmittel-Wissenschaft und -Technologie*, 19: 486–90.

Conner, M.T., Haddon, A.V., Pickering, E.S. and Booth, D.A. (1988b) Sweet tooth demonstrated: individual differences in preference for both sweet foods and foods highly sweetened, *Journal of Applied Psychology*, 73: 275–80.

Conner, M., Martin, E., Silverdale, N. and Grogan, S. (1996) Dieting in adolescence: an application of the theory of planned behaviour, *British Journal of Health Psychology*, 1: 315–25.

Conner, M. and Norman, P. (1994) Comparing the health belief model and the theory of planned behaviour in health screening, in D.R. Rutter and L. Quine (eds) *Social Psychology and Health: European Perspectives*. Aldershot: Avebury.

Conner, M. and Norman, P. (1996) Body weight and shape control: examining component behaviours, *Appetite*, 27: 135–50.

Conner, M., Norman, P. and Bell, R. (2002) The theory of planned behavior and healthy eating, *Health Psychology*, 21: 194–201.

Conner, M., Sheeran, P., Norman, P. and Armitage, C.J. (2000) Temporal stability as a moderator of relationships in the theory of planned behaviour, *British Journal of Social Psychology*, 39: 469–93.

Conner, M. and Sparks, P. (1996) The theory of planned behaviour and health behaviours, in M. Conner and P. Norman (eds) *Predicting Health Behaviour*. Buckingham: Open University Press.

Conner, M. and Sparks, P. (2001) Ambivalence and attitudes, *European Review of Social Psychology*, 12: 37–70.

Conner, M. and Waterman, M. (1996) Questionnaire measures of health-relevant cognitions and behaviours, in J. Haworth (ed.) *Psychological Research: Innovative Methods and Strategies*. London: Routledge.

Cools, J., Schotte, D.E. and McNally, R.J. (1992) Emotional arousal and overeating in restrained eaters, *Journal of Abnormal Psychology*, 101: 348–51.

Cox, D.N., Anderson, A.S., Lean, M.E.J. and Mela, D.J. (1998) UK consumer attitudes, beliefs and barriers to increasing fruit and vegetable consumption, *Public Health Nutrition*, 1: 61–8.

Crandall, C.S. (1994) Prejudice against fat people: Ideology and self-interest, *Journal of Personality and Social Psychology*, 66: 882–94.

Crandall, C.S. (1995) Do parents discriminate against their heavy-weight daughters?, *Personality and Social Psychology Bulletin*, 21: 724–35.

Crandall, C. and Martinez, R. (1996) Culture, ideology, and anti-fat attitudes, *Personality and Social Psychology Bulletin*, 22: 1165–76.

Crisp, A.H., Hsu, L.K.G., Harding, B. and Crowther, J.H. (1980) Clinical features of anorexia nervosa: a study of a consecutive series of 102 female patients, *Journal of Psychosomatic Research*, 24: 179–91.

Crisp, A.H., Palmer, R.L. and Kalucy, R.S. (1976) How common is anorexia nervosa? A prevalence study, *British Journal of Psychiatry*, 128: 549–54.

Crowther, J.H. and Chernyk, B. (1986) Bulimia and binge eating in adolescent females: a comparison, *Addictive Behaviors*, 11: 415–24.

Davison, M. and McCarthy, D. (1988) *The Matching Law: A Research Review*. Hillsdale, NJ: Lawrence Erlbaum Associates.

de Castro, J.M. (1991) Social facilitation of the spontaneous meal size of humans occurs on both weekdays and weekends, *Physiology and Behavior*, 49: 1289–91.

de Castro, J.M. (1994) Family and friends produce greater social facilitation of food intake than other companions, *Physiology and Behavior*, 56: 445–55.

de Castro, J.M. (1997) Socio-cultural determinants of meal size and frequency, *British Journal of Nutrition*, 77: S39–S55.

de Castro, J.M. and Brewer, E.M. (1992) The amount eaten in meals by humans is a power function of the number of people present, *Physiology and Behavior*, 51: 121–5.

de Castro, J.M., Brewer, E.M., Elmore, D.K. and Orozco, S. (1990) Social facilitation of the spontaneous meal size of humans is independent of time, place, alcohol, or snacks, *Appetite*, 15: 89–101.

de Graaf, C., van der Gaag, M., Kafatos, A., Lennernas, M. and Kearney, J.M. (1997) Stages of dietary change among nationally-representative samples of adults in the European Union, *European Journal of Clinical Nutrition*, 51 (Suppl. 2): S47–S56.

Delongis, A., Coyne, J.C., Dakof, G., Folkman, S. and Lazarus, R.S. (1982) Relationship of daily hassles, uplifts and minor life events to health status, *Health Psychology*, 1: 119–36.

Delongis, A., Folkman, S. and Lazarus, R.S. (1984) The impact of daily stress on health and mood: psychological resources as mediators, *Journal of Personality and Social Psychology*, 54, 486–95.

de Luca, R.V. and Spigelman, M.N. (1979) Effects of models on food intake of obese and non-obese college students, *Canadian Journal of Behavioral Science*, 11: 124–9.

Department of Health (DoH) (1992) *The Health of the Nation: A Strategy for Health in England*. London: HMSO.

Department of Health and Human Services (DHHS) (1991) *Healthy People 2000: National Health Promotion and Disease Prevention Objectives*. Washington, DC: DHHS publication PHS 91-50212.

Desor, J.A., Maller, O. and Turner, R.E. (1973) Taste in acceptance of sugars by human infants, *Journal of Comparative and Physiological Psychology*, 84: 496–501.

DiClemente, C.C., Prochaska, J.O., Fairhurst, S.K., *et al.* (1991) The process of smoking cessation: an analysis of precontemplation, contemplation, and preparation stages of change, *Journal of Consulting and Clinical Psychology*, 59: 295–304.

Dijksterhuis, A., Bargh, J.A. and Miedema, J. (2000) Of men and mackerels: attention and automatic behavior, in H. Bless and J.P. Forgas (eds) *Subjective Experience in Social Cognition and Behavior*. Philadelphia: Psychology Press.

Drewnowski, A. (1996) The behavioral phenotype in human obesity, in E.D. Capaldi (ed.) *Why We Eat What We Eat: The Psychology of Eating*. Washington, DC: American Psychological Association.

Dunt, D., Day, N. and Pirkis, J. (1999) Evaluation of a community-based health promotion program supporting public policy initiatives for a healthy diet, *Health Promotion International*, 14: 317–27.

Duran, A. and Trafimow, D. (2000) Cognitive organization of favorable and unfavorable beliefs about performing a behavior, *Journal of Social Psychology*, 140: 179–87.

Eagly, A.H. and Chaiken, S. (1993) *The Psychology of Attitudes*. Fort Worth, TX: Harcourt Brace Jovanovich.

Edwards, W. (1954) The theory of decision making, *Psychological Bulletin*, 51: 380–417.

Ennis, R. and Zanna, M.P. (2000) Attitude function and the automobile, in G.R. Maio and J.M. Olson (eds) *Why We Evaluate: Functions of Attitudes*. London: Lawrence Erlbaum Associates.

Family Heart Study Group (1994) Randomised controlled trial evaluating cardiovascular screening and intervention in general practice: principal results of the British Family Heart study, *British Medical Journal*, 308: 313–20.

Fazio, R.H. (1986) How do attitudes guide behavior?, in R.M. Sorrentino and E.T. Higgins (eds) *Handbook of Motivation and Cognition: Foundations of Social Behavior, Volume 1*. New York: Guilford Press.

Fazio, R.H. (1990) Multiple processes by which attitudes guide behavior: the MODE model as an integrative framework, in M.P. Zanna (ed.) *Advances in Experimental Social Psychology, Volume 23*. San Diego: Academic Press.

Fazio, R.H., Powell, M.C. and Williams, C.J. (1989) The role of attitude accessibility in the attitude-to-behavior process, *Journal of Consumer Research*, 16: 280–8.

Fazio, R.H. and Williams, C.J. (1986) Attitude accessibility as a moderator of the attitude–perception and attitude–behavior relations: an investigation of the 1984 presidential election, *Journal of Personality and Social Psychology*, 51: 505–14.

Fishbein, M. (1967a) A behavior theory approach to the relations between beliefs about an object and the attitude toward the object, in M. Fishbein (ed.) *Readings in Attitude Theory and Measurement*. New York: Wiley.

Fishbein, M. (1967b) Attitude and the prediction of behavior, in M. Fishbein (ed.) *Readings in Attitude Theory and Measurement*. New York: Wiley.

Fishbein, M. (1993) Introduction, in D.J. Terry, C. Gallois and M. McCamish (eds) *The Theory of Reasoned Action: Its Application to AIDS-preventive Behaviour*. Oxford: Pergamon.

Fishbein, M. and Ajzen, I. (1975) *Belief, Attitude, Intention, and Behavior*. New York: Wiley.

Fiske, S.T. and Taylor, S.E. (1991) *Social Cognition*, 2nd edn. New York: McGraw-Hill.

Floyd, D.L., Prentice-Dunn, S. and Rogers, R.W. (2000) A meta-analysis of research on protection motivation theory, *Journal of Applied Social Psychology*, 30: 407–29.

Forkman, B.A. (1991) Social facilitation is shown by gerbils when presented with novel but not with familiar food, *Animal Behaviour*, 42: 860–1.

Fram, E.H. and Cibotti, E. (1991) The shopping list studies and projective techniques: a 40-year view, *Marketing Research*, December: 14–22.

Freeman, S., Walker, M.R., Borden, R. and Latané, B. (1975) Diffusion of responsibility and restaurant tipping: cheaper by the bunch, *Personality and Social Psychology Bulletin*, 1: 584–7.

French, S.A. and Jeffery, R.W. (1994) Consequences of dieting to lose weight: effects on physical and mental health, *Health Psychology*, 13: 195–212.

Fuhrman, A. and Kuhl, J. (1998) Maintaining a healthy diet: effects of personality and self-reward versus self-punishment on commitment to and enactment of self-chosen and assigned goals, *Psychology and Health*, 13: 651–86.

Gallagher, D., Heymsfield, S.B., Heo, M., *et al.* (2000) Healthy percentage body fat ranges: an approach for developing guidelines based on body mass index, *American Journal of Clinical Nutrition*, 72: 694–701.

Gamble, M. and Cotugna, N. (1999) A quarter century of TV food advertising targeted at children, *American Journal of Health Behavior*, 23: 261–7.

Gardner, P., Rosenberg, H.M. and Wilson, R.W. (1996) *Leading Causes of Death by Age, Sex, Race, and Hispanic Origin: United States, 1992*. National Center for Health Statistics, Vital and Health Statistics, 20 (29).

Garfinkel, P.E. and Garner, D.M. (1982) *Anorexia Nervosa: A Multidimensional Perspective*. New York: Brunner/Mazel.

Garner, D., Garfinkel, P., Schwartz, D. and Garfinkel, P. (1980) Cultural expectations of thinness in women, *Psychological Reports*, 47: 483–91.

Garner, D.M. and Bemis, K. (1982) A cognitive behavioural approach to anorexia nervosa, *Cognitive Therapy and Research*, 6: 1–27.

Garrow, J.S. (1977) The regulation of energy expenditure in man, in G.A. Bray (ed.) *Recent Advances in Obesity Research II*. London: Newman.

Geen, R.G. and Gange, J.J. (1977) Drive theory of social facilitation: twelve years of theory and research, *Psychological Bulletin*, 84: 1267–88.

Gelfand, M. (1971) *Diet and Tradition in an African Culture*. London: Livingston Press.

George, L.K. (1989) Stress, social support and depression over the life-course, in K.S. Markides and C.L. Cooper (eds) *Aging, Stress and Health*. New York: Wiley.

Gilbert, S. (1989) Psychological aspects of obesity and its treatment, in R. Shepherd (ed.) *Handbook of the Physiology of Human Eating*. Chichester: Wiley.

Gillman, M.W., Cupples, L.A., Gagnon, D., *et al.* (1995) Protective effect of fruits and vegetables on development of stroke in men, *Journal of the American Medical Association*, 273: 1113–17.

Glanz, K. (1999) Progress in dietary behavior change, *American Journal of Health Promotion*, 14: 112–17.

Godin, G. and Kok, G. (1996) The theory of planned behavior: a review of its applications to health-related behaviors, *American Journal of Health Promotion*, 11: 87–98.

Goldberg, M.E., Gorn, G.J. and Gibson, W. (1978) TV messages for snack and breakfast foods: do they influence children's preferences?, *Journal of Consumer Research*, 5: 73–81.

Gollwitzer, P.M. (1990) Action phases and mind-sets, in E.T. Higgins and R.M. Sorrentino (eds) *Handbook of Motivation and Cognition: Foundations of Social Behavior, Volume 2*. New York: Guilford Press.

Gollwitzer, P.M. (1993) Goal achievement: the role of intentions, *European Review of Social Psychology*, 4: 141–85.

Gollwitzer, P.M. (1996) The volitional benefits of planning, in P.M. Gollwitzer and J.A. Bargh (eds) *The Psychology of Action*. New York: Guilford Press.

Gollwitzer, P. and Bargh, J.A. (eds) (1996) *The Psychology of Action*. New York: Guilford Press.

Gollwitzer, P. and Schall, B. (1998) Metacognition in action: the importance of implementation intentions, *Personality and Social Psychology Review*, 2: 124–36.

Granberg, D. and Holmberg, S. (1990) The intention–behavior relationship among US and Swedish voters, *Social Psychology Quarterly*, 53: 44–54.

Greeno, C.G. and Wing, R.R. (1994) Stress-induced eating, *Psychological Bulletin*, 115: 444–64.

Greenwald, A.G. (1968) Cognitive learning, cognitive response to persuasion, and attitude change, in A.G. Greenwald, T.C. Brock and T.M. Ostrom (eds) *Psychological Foundations of Attitudes*. San Diego: Academic Press.

Greenwald, A.G., McGhee, D.E. and Schwartz, J.L.K. (1998) Measuring individual differences in implicit cognition: the implicit association test, *Journal of Personality and Social Psychology*, 74: 1464–80.

Grogan, S. (1999) *Body Image: Understanding Body Dissatisfaction in Men, Women and Children*. London: Routledge.

Grogan, S. and Cortvreind, P. (submitted) Women's eating: a thematic deconstruction of accounts from women with and without 'eating disorders'.

Grogan, S., Bell, R. and Conner, M. (1997) Eating sweet snack foods: gender differences in attitudes and behaviour, *Appetite*, 28: 19–31.

Grogan, S., Williams, Z. and Conner, M. (1996) An investigation of the effects of viewing attractive same-gender models on body satisfaction, *Psychology of Women Quarterly*, 20: 569–75.

Grunberg, N.E. and Straub, R.O. (1992) The role of gender and taste class in the effects of stress on eating, *Health Psychology*, 11: 97–100.

Haines, H. and Vaughan, G.M. (1979) Was 1898 a great date in the history of social psychology?, *Journal for the History of the Behavioural Sciences*, 15: 323–32.

Haire, M. (1950) Projective techniques in marketing research, *Journal of Marketing*, 19: 649–56.

Harrison, J.A., Mullen, P.D. and Green, L.W. (1992) A meta-analysis of studies of the health belief model with adults, *Health Education Research*, 7: 107–16.

Haslam, C., Stevens, R. and Haslam, R. (1989) Eating habits and stress correlates in a female student population, *Work and Stress*, 3: 327–34.

Hawkins, R.C. and Clement, P.F. (1980) Development and construct validation of a self-report measure of binge eating tendencies, *Addictive Behaviors*, 5: 219–26.

Heald, F.P. (1992) Fast food and snack food: beneficial or deleterious?, *Journal of Adolescent Health*, 13: 380–3.

Heatherton, T.F. and Baumeister, R.F. (1991) Binge eating as an escape from self awareness, *Psychological Bulletin*, 110: 86–108.

Heatherton, T.F., Herman, C.P. and Polivy, J. (1991) Effects of physical threat and ego threat on eating behaviour, *Journal of Personality and Social Psychology*, 60: 138–43.

Heatherton, T.F., Herman, C.P. and Polivy, J. (1992) Effects of distress on eating: the importance of ego-involvement, *Journal of Personality and Social Psychology*, 62: 801–3.

Heatherton, T.F., Striepe, M. and Wittenberg, L. (1998) Emotional control and dis-inhibited eating: the role of self, *Personality and Social Psychology Bulletin*, 24: 301–13.

Heckhausen, H. (1991) *Motivation and Action*. Berlin: Springer.

Helweg-Larsen, M. and Shepperd, J.A. (2001) Do moderators of the optimistic bias affect personal or target risk estimates? A review of the literature, *Personality and Social Psychology Review*, 5: 74–95.

Herman, C.P. (1978) Restrained eating, *Psychiatric Clinics of North America*, 1: 593–607.

Herman, C.P. and Mack, D. (1975) Restrained and unrestrained eating, *Journal of Personality*, 43: 647–60.

Herman, C.P. and Polivy, J. (1975) Anxiety, restraint, and eating behavior, *Journal of Abnormal Psychology*, 84: 666–72.

Herrnstein, R.J. (1961) Relative and absolute strength of response as a function of fre-
quency of reinforcement, *Journal of the Experimental Analysis of Behavior*, 4: 267–72.
Herrnstein, R.J. (1970) On the law of effect, *Journal of the Experimental Analysis of
Behavior*, 13: 243–66.
Hill, A.J., Oliver, S. and Rogers, P.J. (1992) Eating in the adult world: the rise of dieting
in childhood and adolescence, *British Journal of Clinical Psychology*, 31: 95–105.
Hill, A.J., Weaver, C.F.L. and Blundell, J.E. (1991) Food craving, dietary restraint and
mood, *Appetite*, 17: 187–97.
Hitchings, E. and Moynihan, P.J. (1998) The relationship between television food
advertisements recalled and actual foods consumed by children, *Journal of Human
Nutrition and Dietetics*, 11: 511–17.
Holland, A.J., Hall, A., Murray, R., Russell, G.F.M. and Crisp, A.H. (1984) Anorexia
nervosa: a study of 34 twin pairs and one set of triplets, *British Journal of Psychiatry*,
145: 414–19.
Holmes, T.J. and Rahe, R.H. (1967) The social readjustment rating scale. *Journal of
Psychosomatic Research*, 11: 213–18.
Houston, D.A. and Fazio, R.H. (1989) Biased processing as a function of attitude
accessibility: making objective judgements subjectively, *Social Cognition*, 7: 51–66.
Howard-Pitney, B., Winkleby, M.A., Albright, C.L., Bruce, B. and Fortmann, S.P. (1997)
The Stanford Nutrition Action Program: a dietary fat intervention for low-literacy
adults, *American Journal of Public Health*, 87: 1971–6.
Howell, D.C. (1992) *Statistical Methods for Psychology*, 3rd edn. Belmont, CA: Duxbury
Press.
International Obesity Task Force (2001) About obesity (www.obesity.chair.ulaval.ca/
IOTF.htm).
Itzin, C. (1986) Media images of women: the social construction of ageism and sexism,
in S. Wilkinson (ed.) *Feminist Social Psychology*. Milton Keynes: Open University
Press.
Jacobs, D.R., Marquart, L., Slavin, J. and Kushi, L.H. (1998) Whole-grain intake and
cancer: an expanded review and meta-analysis, *Nutrition and Cancer*, 30: 85–96.
Janis, I.L., and Feshbach, S. (1953) Effects of fear-arousing communications, *Journal of
Abnormal and Social Psychology*, 48: 403–10.
Janis, I.L. and Mann, L. (1977) *Decision Making: A Psychological Analysis of Conflict,
Choice and Commitment*. New York: The Free Press.
Janz, N. and Becker, M.H. (1984) The health belief model: a decade later, *Health
Education Quarterly*, 11: 1–47.
Jeffery, R.W., Drewnowski, A., Epstein, L.H., *et al.* (2000) Long-term maintenance of
weight loss: current status, *Health Psychology*, 19: 5–16.
Jequier, E. (1987) Energy utilization in human obesity, in R.J. Wurtman and J.J. Wurtman
(eds) *Human Obesity*. New York: New York Academy of Sciences.
Johar, J.S. and Sirgy, M.J. (1991) Value-expressive versus utilitarian advertising appeals:
when and why to use which appeal, *Journal of Advertising*, 20: 23–33.
Johnson, B.T. and Eagly, A.H. (1989) Effects of involvement on persuasion: a meta-
analysis, *Psychological Bulletin*, 106: 290–314.
Johnson-Sabine, E., Reiss, D. and Dayson, D. (1982) Bulimia nervosa: a 5-year follow-
up study, *Psychological Medicine*, 22: 951–9.
Joshipura, K.J., Ascherio, A., Manson, J.E., *et al.* (1999) Fruit and vegetable intake in
relation to risk of ischemic stroke, *Journal of the American Medical Association*, 282:
1233–9.

Kaplan, H.I. and Kaplan, H.S. (1957) The psychosomatic concept of obesity, *Journal of Nervous and Mental Disorders*, 125: 181–201.

Katz, D. (1960) The functional approach to the study of attitudes, *Public Opinion Quarterly*, 24: 163–204.

Kaye, W.H., Klump, K.L., Frank, G.K.W. and Stober, M. (2000) Anorexia and bulimia nervosa, *Annual Review of Medicine*, 51: 299–313.

Kendzierski, D. (1990) Decision making versus decision implementation: an action control approach to exercise adoption and adherence, *Journal of Applied Social Psychology*, 20: 27–45.

Keys, A. (1980) *Seven Countries: A Multivariate Analysis of Death and Coronary Heart Disease*. Cambridge, MA: Harvard University Press.

Kim, M.-S. and Hunter, J.E. (1993) Attitude-behavior relations: a meta-analysis of attitudinal relevance and topic, *Journal of Communication*, 43: 101–42.

Kraus, S.J. (1995) Attitudes and the prediction of behavior: a meta-analysis of the empirical literature, *Personality and Social Psychology Bulletin*, 21: 58–75.

Kreuter, M.W. and Skinner, C.S. (2000) Tailoring: what's in a name?, *Health Education Research*, 15: 1–4.

Kristal, A.R., Glanz, K., Tilley, B.C. and Li, S. (2000) Mediating factors in dietary change: understanding the impact of a nutrition intervention, *Health Education and Behavior*, 27: 112–25.

Kuczmarski, R.J., Flegal, K.M., Campbell, S.M. and Johnson, C.L. (1994) Increasing prevalence of overweight among US adults: the National Health and Nutrition Examination Surveys, 1960 to 1991, *JAMA: Journal of the American Medical Association*, 272: 205–11.

Kuhl, J. (1985) Volitional mediators of cognition–behavior consistency: self-regulatory processes and action versus state orientation, in J. Kuhl and J. Beckman (eds) *Action Control: From Cognition to Behavior*. New York: Springer.

Kuhl, J. and Beckman, J. (1985) *Action Control: From Cognition to Behavior*. New York: Springer.

Kumanyika, S.K., van Horn, L., Bowen, D., *et al.* (2000) Maintenance of dietary behavior change, *Health Psychology*, 19 (Suppl.): 42–56.

Lacey, J.H., Coker, S. and Birtchnell, S.A. (1986) Bulimia: Factors associated with its etiology and maintenance, *International Journal of Eating Disorders*, 5: 475–87.

Laforge, R.G., Velicer, W.F., Richmond, R.L. and Owen, N. (1999) Stage distributions for five health behaviors in the United States and Australia, *Preventive Medicine*, 28: 61–74.

Lamb, C.S., Jackson, L., Cassiday, P. and Priest, D. (1993) Body figure preferences of men and women: A comparison of two generations, *Gender Roles*, 28: 345–58.

Latané, B. (1981) The psychology of social impact, *American Psychologist*, 36: 343–55.

Law, M.R., Frost, C.D. and Wald, N.J. (1991) By how much does dietary salt lower blood pressure? I – Analysis of observational data among populations, *British Medical Journal*, 302: 811–15.

Law, M.R. and Morris, J.K. (1998) By how much does fruit and vegetable consumption reduce the risk of ischaemic heart disease?, *European Journal of Clinical Nutrition*, 52: 549–56.

Lazarus, R.S. and Folkman, S. (1984) *Stress, Appraisal and Coping*. New York: Springer.

Lewis, M.K. and Hill, A.J. (1998) Food advertising on British children's television: a content analysis and experimental study with nine-year olds, *International Journal of Obesity*, 22: 206–14.

Linden, J., Gregorio, D. and Kalish, R. (1988) An estimate of the blood donor eligibility in the general population, *Vox Sanguinis*, 54: 96–100.

Lissner, L., Odell, P.M., D'Agostino, R.B., *et al.* (1991) Variability of body weight and health outcomes in the Framingham population, *New England Journal of Medicine*, 324: 1839–44.

Logue, A.W. (1991) *The Psychology of Eating and Drinking*, 2nd edn. New York: Freeman.

Lowe, M.R. (1993) The effects of dieting on eating behavior: a three factor model, *Psychological Bulletin*, 114: 100–21.

Lozano, D.I., Crites, S.L. and Aikman, S.N. (1999) Changes in food attitudes as a function of hunger, *Appetite*, 32: 207–18.

McAuley, E. (1993) Self-efficacy and the maintenance of exercise participation in older adults, *Journal of Behavioral Medicine*, 15: 65–88.

Maccoby, N., Farquhar, J.W., Wood, P.D. and Alexander, J. (1977) Reducing the risk of cardiovascular disease: effects of a community-based campaign on knowledge and behavior, *Journal of Community Health*, 3: 100–14.

MacDougall, D.B. (1987) Effects of pigmentation, light scatter and illumination on food appearance and acceptance, in J. Solms, D.A. Booth, R.M. Pangborn and O. Raunhardt (eds) *Food Acceptance and Nutrition*. London: Academic Press.

Macrae, C.N. and Johnston, L. (1998) Help, I need somebody: automatic action and inaction, *Social Cognition*, 16: 400–17.

McCrae, R.R. and John, O.P. (1992) An introduction to the five-factor model and its applications, *Journal of Personality*, 60: 175–215.

Manstead, A.S.R. and Parker, D. (1995) Evaluating and extending the theory of planned behaviour, in W. Stroebe and M. Hewstone (eds) *European Review of Social Psychology, Volume 6*. Chichester: Wiley.

Manstead, A.S.R. and Semin, G. (1996) Methodology in social psychology: Putting ideas to the test, in M. Hewstone, W. Stroebe and G.M. Stephenson (eds) *Introduction to Social Psychology*. London: Blackwell.

Marcus, B.H., Dubbert, P.M., Forsyth, L.H., *et al.* (2000) Physical activity behavior change: Issues in adoption and maintenance, *Health Psychology*, 19: 32–41.

Marcus, B.H., Rossi, J.S., Selby, V.C., Niaura, R.S. and Abrams, D.B. (1992) The stages and processes of exercise adoption and maintenance in a worksite sample, *Health Psychology*, 11: 257–61.

Margetts, B.M., Cade, J.E. and Osmond, C. (1989) Comparison of a food frequency questionnaire with a diet record, *International Journal of Epidemiology*, 18: 868–73.

Marlatt, G.A. and Gordon, J. (eds) (1985) *Relapse Prevention: Maintenance Strategies in Addictive Behavior Change*. New York: Guilford Press.

Martin, M.J., Hulley, S.B., Browner, W.S., Kuller, L.H. and Wentworth, D. (1986) Serum cholesterol, blood pressure, and mortality: implications from a cohort of 361,662 men, *The Lancet*, 8513: 833–9.

Mendelson, B.K. and White, D.R. (1982) Relation between body-esteem of obese and normal children, *Perceptual and Motor Skills*, 54: 899–905.

Metropolitan Life Insurance Company (1983) 1983 metropolitan height and weight tables, *Statistical Bulletin of the Metropolitan Life Insurance Company*, 64: 2.

Michaud, C., Kahn, J.P., Musse, N., *et al.* (1990) Relationships between a critical life event and eating behaviour in high-school students, *Stress Medicine*, 6: 57–64.

Miller, L., Rozin, P. and Fiske, A.P. (1998) Food sharing and feeding another person suggests intimacy: two studies of American college students, *European Journal of Social Psychology*, 28: 423–36.

Milne, S., Sheeran, P. and Orbell, S. (2000) Prediction and intervention in health-related behavior: a meta-analytic review of protection motivation theory, *Journal of Applied Social Psychology*, 30: 106–43.

Mischel, W., Shoda, Y. and Rodriguez, M.L. (1989) Delay of gratification in children. *Science*, 244: 933–8.

Mistiaen, V. (1997) Take a pass on the fish sticks, *Chicago Tribune*, 6 April, Section 13.

Mori, D., Chaiken, S. and Pliner, P. (1987) 'Eating lightly' and the self-presentation of femininity, *Journal of Personality and Social Psychology*, 53: 693–702.

Mullen, P.D., Hersey, J.C. and Iverson, D.C. (1987) Health behavior models compared, *Social Science and Medicine*, 24: 973–83.

Mussell, M.P., Binford, R.B. and Fulkerson, J.A. (2000) Eating disorders: summary of risk factors, prevention programming, and prevention research, *Counselling Psychology*, 28: 764–96.

Nemeroff, C. and Rozin, P. (1989) An unacknowledged belief that 'you are what you eat' among college students in the United States: an application of the demand free 'impressions' technique, *Ethos: The Journal of Psychological Anthropology*, 17: 50–69.

Netemeyer, R.G., Burton, S. and Johnston, M. (1991) A comparison of two models for the prediction of volitional and goal-directed behaviors: a confirmatory analysis approach, *Social Psychology Quarterly*, 54: 87–100.

Nguyen, M.N., Otis, J. and Potvin, L. (1996) Determinants of intention to adopt a low-fat diet in men 30 to 60 years old: implications for heart health promotions, *American Journal of Health Promotion*, 10: 201–7.

Nisbett, R.E. (1972) Hunger, obesity, and the ventromedial hypothalamus, *Psychological Review*, 79: 433–53.

Nisbett, R.E. and Storms, M.D. (1974) Cognitive and social determinants of food intake, in H. London and R.E. Nisbett (eds) *Thought and Feeling: Cognitive Alteration of Feeling States*. Chicago: Aldine.

O'Brien, T.B. and Delongis, A. (1996) The interactional context of problem-, emotion-, and relationship-focused coping: the role of the big five personality factors, *Journal of Personality*, 64: 775–811.

Obrist, P.A. (1981) *Cardiovascular Psychophysiology: A Perspective*. New York: Plenum.

Oliver, G. and Wardle, J. (1999) Perceived effects of stress on food choice, *Physiology and Behavior*, 66: 511–15.

Oliver, G., Wardle, J. and Gibson, L. (2000) Stress and food choice: a laboratory study, *Psychosomatic Medicine*, 62: 853–65.

Olsen, S.O. (1999) Strength and conflicting valence in the measurement of food attitudes and preferences, *Food Quality and Preference*, 10: 483–94.

Orbach, S. (1993) *Hunger Strike: The Anorectic's Struggle as a Metaphor for Our Age*. London: Penguin.

Ouellette, J.A. and Wood, W. (1998) Habit and intention in everyday life: the multiple processes by which past behavior predicts future behavior, *Psychological Bulletin*, 124: 54–74.

Owen, W.P., Halmi, K.A., Gibbs, J. and Smith, G.P. (1985) Satiety responses in eating disorders, *Journal of Psychiatric Research*, 19: 279–84.

OXCHECK Study Group (1994) Effectiveness of health checks conducted by nurses in primary care: results of the OXCHECK study after one year, *British Medical Journal*, 308: 308–12.

Paisley, C.M. and Sparks, P. (1998) Expectations of reducing fat intake: the role of perceived need within the theory of planned behaviour, *Psychology and Health*, 13: 341–53.

Parker, D., Manstead, A.S.R. and Stradling, S.G. (1995) Extending the theory of planned behaviour: the role of personal norm, *British Journal of Social Psychology*, 34: 127–37.

Peak, H. (1955) Attitude and motivation, in M.R. Jones (ed.) *Nebraska Symposium on Motivation*. Lincoln: University of Nebraska Press.

Pelchat, M.L. and Rozin, P. (1982) The special role of nausea in the acquisition of food dislikes by humans, *Appetite*, 3: 341–51.

Perri, M.G., Nezu, A.M., Patti, E.T. and McCann, K.L. (1989) Effect of length of treatment on weight loss, *Journal of Consulting and Clinical Psychology*, 57: 450–2.

Perugini, M. and Conner, M. (2000) Predicting and understanding behavioral volitions: the interplay between goals and behaviors, *European Journal of Social Psychology*, 30: 705–31.

Petty, R.E. and Cacioppo, J.T. (1986) *Communication and Persuasion: Central and Peripheral Routes to Attitude Change*. New York: Springer.

Pine, C.J. (1985) Anxiety and eating behaviour in obese and non-obese American Indians and white Americans, *Journal of Personality and Social Psychology*, 49: 774–80.

Pliner, P. and Chaiken, S. (1990) Eating, social motives, and self-presentation in women and men, *Journal of Experimental Social Psychology*, 26: 240–54.

Pliner, P., Chaiken, S. and Flett, G.L. (1990) Gender differences in concern with body weight and physical appearance over the life span, *Personality and Social Psychology Bulletin*, 16: 263–73.

Plotnikoff, R.C. and Higginbotham, N. (1995) Predicting low-fat diet intentions and behaviors for the prevention of coronary heart disease: an application of protection motivation theory among an Australian population, *Psychology and Health*, 10: 397–408.

Pope, H.G., Hudson, J.I., Jonas, J.M. and Yurgelun-Todd, D. (1983) Bulimia treated with imipramine: a placebo-controlled, double-blind study, *American Journal of Psychiatry*, 140: 554–8.

Povey, R., Conner, M., Sparks, P., James, R. and Shepherd, R. (1998) Interpretations of healthy and unhealthy eating, and implications for dietary change, *Health Education Research*, 13: 171–83.

Povey, R., Conner, M., Sparks, P., James, R. and Shepherd, R. (2000) Application of the theory of planned behaviour to two dietary behaviours: roles of perceived control and self-efficacy, *British Journal of Health Psychology*, 5: 121–39.

Povey, R., Wellens, B. and Conner, M. (2001) Attitudes towards following meat, vegetarian and vegan diets: an examination of the role of ambivalence, *Appetite*, 37: 15–26.

Powell, M.C. and Fazio, R.H. (1984) Attitude accessibility as a function of repeated expression, *Personality and Social Psychology Bulletin*, 10: 139–48.

Powley, T.L. (1977) The ventromedial hypothalamic syndrome, satiety, and a cephalic phase hypothesis, *Psychological Review*, 84: 89–126.

Prevost, A.T., Whichelow, M.J. and Cox, B.D. (1997) Longitudinal dietary changes between 1984–5 and 1991–2 in British adults: associations with socio-demographics, lifestyle and health factors, *British Journal of Nutrition*, 78: 873–88.

Price, R.A. and Stunkard, A.J. (1989) Commingling analysis of obesity in twins, *Human Heredity*, 39: 121–35.

Prochaska, J.O. (1979) *Systems of Psychotherapy: A Transtheoretical Analysis*. Homewood, IL: Dorsey Press.

Prochaska, J.O. and DiClemente, C.C. (1983) Stages and processes of self-change in smoking: toward an integrative model of change, *Journal of Consulting and Clinical Psychology*, 51: 390–5.

Prochaska, J.O. and DiClemente, C.C. (1984) *The Transtheoretical Approach: Crossing the Traditional Boundaries of Change*. Homewood, IL: J. Irwin.

Prochaska, J.O. and DiClemente, C.C. (1986) Toward a comprehensive model of change, in W.R. Miller and N. Heather (eds) *Treating Addictive Behaviors: Processes of Change*. New York: Plenum Press.

Prochaska, J.O., DiClemente, C.C. and Norcross, J.C. (1992) In search of how people change: applications to addictive behaviors, *American Psychologist*, 47: 1102–14.

Prochaska, J.O., Redding, C.A., Harlow, L.L., Rossi, J.S. and Velicer, W.F. (1994a) The transtheoretical model of change and HIV prevention: a review, *Health Education Quarterly*, 21: 471–86.

Prochaska, J.O., Velicer, W.F., Rossi, J.S., *et al.* (1994b) Stages of change and decisional balance for 12 problem behaviors, *Health Psychology*, 13: 39–46.

Pulliam, H.R. (1974) On the theory of optimal diets, *American Naturalist*, 108: 59–74.

Ramsay, L.E., Yeo, W.W. and Jackson, P.R. (1991) Dietary reduction of serum cholesterol concentration: time to think again, *British Medical Journal*, 303: 953.

Randall, E. and Sanjur, D. (1981) Food preferences: their conceptualization and relationship to consumption, *Ecology of Food and Nutrition*, 11: 151–61.

Ravussin, E., Lillioja, S., Knowler, W.C., *et al.* (1988) Reduced rate of energy expenditure as a risk factor for body weight gain, *New England Journal of Medicine*, 318: 467–72.

Redd, M. and de Castro, J.M. (1992) Social facilitation of eating: effects of social instruction on food intake, *Physiology and Behavior*, 52: 749–54.

Reger, B., Wootan, M.G. and Booth-Butterfield, S. (1999) Using mass media to promote healthy eating: a community-based demonstration project, *Preventive Medicine*, 29: 414–21.

Resnicow, K., Davis-Hearn, M., Smith, M., *et al.* (1997) Social-cognitive predictors of fruit and vegetable intake in children, *Health Psychology*, 16: 272–6.

Richard, R., de Vries, N. and van der Pligt, J. (1998) Anticipated regret and precautionary sexual behavior, *Journal of Applied Social Psychology*, 28: 1411–1428.

Richard, R., van der Pligt, J. and de Vries, N. (1995) Anticipated affective reactions and prevention of AIDS, *British Journal of Social Psychology*, 34: 9–21.

Richard, R., van der Pligt, J. and de Vries, N. (1996) Anticipated affect and behavioral choice, *Basic and Applied Social Psychology*, 18: 111–29.

Richins, M. (1991) Social comparison and the idealized images of advertising, *Journal of Consumer Research*, 18: 71–83.

Robbins, T.W. and Fray, P.J. (1980) Stress induced eating – fact, fiction or misunderstanding, *Appetite*, 1: 103–33.

Rodin, J. (1981) The externality theory today, in A.J. Stunkard (ed.) *Obesity*. Philadelphia: W.B. Saunders.

Rogers, P.J. and Blundell, J.E. (1990) Psychobiological bases of food choice, *British Nutrition Foundation Nutrition Bulletin*, 15 (Suppl. 1): 31–40.

Rogers, R.W. (1983) Cognitive and physiological processes in fear appeals and attitude change: a revised theory of protection motivation, in J. Cacioppo and R. Petty (eds) *Social Psychophysiology*. New York: Guilford Press.

Rolls, B.J., Rolls, E.T., Rowe, E.A. and Sweeney, K. (1981) Sensory specific satiety in man, *Physiology and Behavior*, 27: 137–42.

Rolls, B.J., van Duijenvoorde, P.M. and Rolls, E.T. (1984) Pleasantness changes and food intake in a varied four-course meal, *Appetite*, 5: 337–48.

Rose, G. (1985) Sick individuals and sick populations, *International Journal of Epidemiology*, 14: 32–8.

Rosen, J.C., Compas, B.E. and Tacy, B. (1993) The relation among stress, psychological symptoms, and eating disorder symptoms: a prospective analysis, *International Journal of Eating Disorders*, 14: 153–62.

Rosen, J.C., Tacy, B. and Howell, D. (1990) Life stress, psychological symptoms and weight reducing behavior in adolescent girls: a prospective analysis, *International Journal of Eating Disorders*, 9: 17–26.

Rosenberg, M.J. and Hovland, C.I. (1960) Cognitive, affective, and behavioral components of attitudes, in C.I. Hovland and M.J. Rosenberg (eds) *Attitude Organization and Change: An Analysis of Consistency among Attitude Components*. New Haven, CT: Yale University Press.

Rosenstock, I.M. (1974) Historical origins of the health belief model, *Health Education Monographs*, 2: 1–8.

Roth, D.A., Herman, C.P., Polivy, J. and Pliner, P. (2001) Self-presentational conflict in social eating situations: a normative perspective, *Appetite*, 36, 165–71.

Rothblum, E. (1990) Women and weight: fad and fiction, *Journal of Psychology*, 124: 5–24.

Rothman, A.J. (2000) Toward a theory-based analysis of behavioral maintenance, *Health Psychology*, 19: 64–9.

Rozin, P. (1990) The importance of social factors in understanding the acquisition of food habits, in E.D. Capaldi and T.L Powley (eds) *Taste, Experience, and Feeding*. Washington, DC: American Psychological Association.

Rozin, P., Ashmore, M. and Markwith, M. (1996) Lay American conceptions of nutrition: dose insensitivity, categorical thinking, contagion, and the monotonic mind, *Health Psychology*, 15, 438–47.

Rozin, P. and Fallon, A.E. (1981) The acquisition of likes and dislikes for foods, in J. Solms and R.L. Hall (eds) *Criteria of Food Acceptance: How Man Chooses What He Eats. A Symposium*. Zurich: Forster.

Rozin, P. and Fallon, A.E. (1987) A perspective on disgust, *Psychological Review*, 94: 23–41.

Rozin, P. and Vollmecke, T. (1986) Food likes and dislikes, *Annual Review of Nutrition*, 6: 433–56.

Russell, G.F.M., Szmukler, G.I., Dare, C. and Eisler, I. (1987) An evaluation of family therapy in anorexia nervosa and bulimia nervosa, *Archives of General Psychiatry*, 44: 1047–56.

Rutter, D.R. and Quine, L. (eds) (2002) *Changing Health Behaviour: Intervention and Research with Social Cognition Models*. Buckingham: Open University Press.

Ryckman, R.M., Robbins, M.A., Kaczor, L.M. and Gold, J.A. (1989) Male and female raters' stereotyping of male and female physiques, *Personality and Social Psychology Bulletin*, 15: 244–51.

Sanbonmatsu, D.M. and Fazio, R.H. (1990) The role of attitudes in memory-based decision making, *Journal of Personality and Social Psychology*, 59: 614–22.

Sandman, P.M. and Weinstein, N.D. (1993) Predictors of home radon testing an implications for testing promotion programs, *Health Education Quarterly*, 20: 471–87.

Sapp, S.G. and Jensen, H.H. (1998) An evaluation of the health belief model for predicting perceived and actual dietary quality, *Journal of Applied Social Psychology*, 28: 235–48.

Saunders, R.P. and Rahilly, S.A. (1990) Influences on intention to reduce dietary intake of fat and sugar, *Journal of Nutrition Education*, 22: 169–76.

Schachter, S. (1971) Some extraordinary facts about obese humans and rats, *American Psychologist*, 26: 129–44.

Schachter, S., Goldman, R. and Gordon, A. (1968) Effects of fear, food deprivation and obesity on eating, *Journal of Personality and Social Psychology*, 10: 91–7.

Schafer, R.B., Keith, P.M. and Schafer, E. (1995) Predicting fat in diets of marital partners using the health belief model, *Journal of Behavioral Medicine*, 18: 419–33.

Schifter, D.B. and Ajzen, I. (1985) Intention, perceived control, and weight loss: an application of the theory of planned behavior, *Journal of Personality and Social Psychology*, 49: 843–51.

Schlundt, D.G., Taylor, D., Hill, J.O., *et al.* (1991) A behavioral taxonomy of obese female participants in a weight loss program, *American Journal of Clinical Nutrition*, 53: 1151–8.

Schneider, D.J. (1991) Social cognition, *Annual Review of Psychology*, 42: 527–61.

Schotte, D.E., Cools, J. and McNally, R.J. (1990) Film-induced negative affect triggers overeating in restrained eaters, *Journal of Abnormal Psychology*, 99: 317–20.

Schuette, R.A. and Fazio, R.H. (1995) Attitude accessibility and motivation as determinants of biased processing – a test of the MODE model, *Personality and Social Psychology Bulletin*, 21: 704–10.

Schuler, G., Hambrecht, R., Schlierf, G., *et al.* (1992) Regular physical exercise and low-fat diet: effects on progression of coronary artery disease, *Circulation*, 86: 1–11.

Schutz, H.G. and Diaz-Knauf, K.V. (1989) The role of the mass media in influencing eating, in R. Shepherd (ed.) *Handbook of the Physiology of Human Eating*. Chichester: Wiley.

Schwartz, R.S., Ravussin, E., Massari, M., O'Connell, M. and Robbins, D.C. (1985) The thermic effect of carbohydrate versus fat feeding in man, *Metabolism*, 34: 285–93.

Schwarzer, R. (1992) Self-efficacy in the adoption and maintenance of health behaviors: theoretical approaches and a new model, in R. Schwarzer (ed.) *Self-efficacy: Thought Control of Action*. Washington, DC: Hemisphere.

Schwarzer, R. and Fuchs, R. (1996) Self-efficacy and health behaviours, in M. Conner and P. Norman (eds) *Predicting Health Behaviour*. Buckingham: Open University Press.

Schwarzer, R. and Renner, B. (2000) Social-cognitive predictors of health behavior: action self-efficacy and coping self-efficacy, *Health Psychology*, 19: 487–95.

Sejwacz, D., Ajzen, I. and Fishbein, M. (1980) Predicting and understanding weight loss, in I. Ajzen and M. Fishbein (eds) *Understanding Attitudes and Predicting Social Behavior*. Englewood Cliffs, NJ: Prentice Hall.

Shannon, B., Bagby, R., Wang, M.Q. and Trenkner, L. (1990) Self-efficacy: a contributor to the explanation of eating behavior, *Health Education Research*, 5: 395–407.

Shavitt, S. (1990) The role of attitude objects in attitude functions, *Journal of Experimental Social Psychology*, 26: 124–48.

Shavitt, S. and Fazio, R.H. (1991) Effects of attribute salience on the consistency between attitudes and behavior predictions, *Personality and Social Psychology Bulletin*, 17: 507–16.

Shavitt, S., Lowrey, T.M. and Han, S. (1992) Attitude functions in advertising: the interactive role of products and self-monitoring, *Journal of Consumer Psychology*, 1: 337–64.

Sheeran, P. (2002) Intention–behaviour relations: a conceptual and empirical review, *European Review of Social Psychology*, 12: 1–36.

Sheeran, P. and Abraham, C. (1996) The health belief model, in M. Conner and P. Norman (eds) *Predicting Health Behaviour*. Buckingham: Open University Press.

Sheeshka, J.D., Woolcott, D.M. and MacKinnon, N.J. (1993) Social cognitive theory as a framework to explain intentions to practice healthy eating behaviors, *Journal of Applied Social Psychology*, 23: 1547–73.

Sheiham, A., Marmot, M., Rawson, D. and Ruck, N. (1987) Food values: health and diet, in R. Jowell, S. Witherspoon and L. Brook (eds) *British Social Attitudes: The 1987 Report*. London: Gower, Social and Community Planning Research.

Shepherd, R. (1989) Factors influencing food preferences and choice, in R. Shepherd (ed.) *Handbook of the Physiology of Human Eating*. Chichester: Wiley.

Shepherd, R. (1999) Social determinants of food choice, *Proceedings of the Nutrition Society*, 58: 807–12.

Shepherd, R. and Farleigh, C.A. (1989) Sensory assessment of foods and the role of sensory attributes in determining food choice, in R. Shepherd (ed.) *Handbook of the Physiology of Human Eating*. Chichester: Wiley.

Sheppard, B.H., Hartwick, J. and Warshaw, P.R. (1988) The theory of reasoned action: a meta-analysis of past research with recommendations for modifications and future research, *Journal of Consumer Research*, 15: 325–43.

Sherif, M. (1936) *The Psychology of Social Norms*. New York: Harper and Bros.

Shu, X.O., Zheng, W., Potischman, N., *et al.* (1993) A population-based case–control study of dietary factors and endometrial cancer in Shanghai, People's Republic of China, *American Journal of Epidemiology*, 137: 155–65.

Silverstein, B., Peterson, B. and Purdue, L. (1986) Some correlates of the then standard of physical attractiveness of women, *International Journal of Eating Disorders*, 5: 898–905.

Simonson, I. (1992) The influence of anticipating regret and responsibility on purchase decisions, *Journal of Consumer Research*, 19: 105–18.

Smith, J. (1996) *Hungry for You. From Cannibalism to Seduction: A Book of Food*. London: Chatto and Windus.

Smith, J. (2002) *Psychology of Food*. Basingstoke: Palgrave.

Sobal, J. and Stunkard, A.J. (1989) Socioeconomic status and obesity: a review of the literature, *Psychological Bulletin*, 105: 260–75.

Sommer, R. and Steele, J. (1997) Social effects on duration in restaurants, *Appetite*, 29: 25–30.

Sparks, P. (1994) Attitudes towards food: applying, assessing and extending the 'theory of planned behaviour', in D.R. Rutter and L. Quine (eds) *Social Psychology and Health: European Perspectives*. Aldershot: Avebury Press.

Sparks, P. (2000) Subjective expected utility-based attitude–behavior models: the utility of self-identity, in D.J. Terry and M.A. Hogg (eds) *Attitudes, Behavior and Social Context: The Role of Norms and Group Membership*. London: Lawrence Erlbaum.

Sparks, P., Conner, M., James, R., Povey, R. and Shepherd, R. (1996) Problems, plans and precommitments, in E. Nyhus and S.V. Troye (eds) *Frontiers in Economic Psychology, Volume II*. Bergen: IAREP/NHH.

Sparks, P., Conner, M., James, R., Shepherd, R. and Povey, R. (2001) Ambivalence about health-related behaviours: an exploration in the domain of food choice, *British Journal of Health Psychology*, 6: 53–68.

Sparks, P. and Guthrie, C.A. (1998) Self-identity and the theory of planned behavior: a useful addition or unhelpful artifice?, *Journal of Applied Social Psychology*, 28: 1394–411.

Sparks, P., Hedderley, D. and Shepherd, R. (1992) An investigation into the relationship between perceived control, attitude variability and the consumption of two common foods, *European Journal of Social Psychology*, 22: 55–71.

Sparks, P. and Shepherd, R. (1992) Self-identity and the theory of planned behavior – assessing the role of identification with green consumerism, *Social Psychology Quarterly*, 55: 388–99.

Sparks, P., Shepherd, R. and Frewer, L.J. (1995) Assessing and structuring attitudes toward the use of gene technology in food production: the role of perceived ethical obligation, *Basic and Applied Social Psychology*, 16: 267–85.

Spillman, D. (1990) Survey of food and vitamin intake responses reported by university students experiencing stress, *Psychological Reports*, 66: 499–502.

Spitzer, L. and Rodin, J. (1981) Human eating behavior: a critical review of studies in normal weight and overweight individuals, *Appetite*, 2: 293–329.

Stallones, R.A. (1983) Ischemic heart disease and lipids in blood and diet, *Annual Review of Nutrition*, 3: 155–85.

Stamler, J., Wentworth, D. and Neaton, J.D. (1986) Is relationship between serum cholesterol and risk of premature death from coronary heart disease continuous and graded? Findings in 356,222 primary screenees of the Multiple Risk Factor Intervention Trial (MRFIT), *Journal of the American Medical Association*, 256: 2823–8.

Stein, R.I. and Nemeroff, C.J. (1995) Moral overtones of food: judgments of others based on what they eat, *Personality and Social Psychology Bulletin*, 21: 480–90.

Steiner, J.E. (1977) Facial expressions of the neonate infant indicating the hedonics of food-related chemical stimuli, in J.M. Weiffenbach (ed.) *Taste and Development: The Genesis of Sweet Preference*. Washington, DC: US Government Printing Office.

Steiner, J.E. (1979) Human facial expressions in response to taste and smell stimulation, *Advances in Child Development*, 13: 257–95.

Steptoe, A., Doherty, S., Rink, E., *et al.* (1999) Behavioural counselling in general practice for the promotion of health behaviour among adults at increased risk of coronary heart disease: randomised trial, *British Medical Journal*, 319: 943–8.

Steptoe, A., Lipsey, Z. and Wardle, J. (1998) Stress, hassles and variations in alcohol consumption, food choice and physical exercise: a diary study, *British Journal of Health Psychology*, 3: 51–63.

Stice, E. (1994) Review of the evidence for a sociocultural model of bulimia nervosa and an exploration of the mechanisms of action, *Clinical Psychology Review*, 14: 633–61.

Stone, A.A. and Brownell, K.D. (1994) The stress-eating paradox. Multiple daily measurements in adult males and females, *Psychology and Health*, 9: 425–36.

Stone, A.A. and Neal, J.M. (1984) A new measure of daily coping: development and preliminary results, *Journal of Personality and Social Psychology*, 46: 892–906.

Stulb, S.C., McDonough, J.R., Greenberg, B.G. and Hames, C.G. (1965) The relationship of nutrient intake and exercise to serum cholesterol level in white males in Evans County, Georgia, *American Journal of Clinical Nutrition*, 16: 238–42.

Stunkard, A.J. (1959) Eating patterns and obesity, *Psychiatric Quarterly*, 33: 284–92.

Stunkard, A.J. (1982) Obesity, in A.S. Bellack, M. Hersen and A.E. Kazdin (eds) *International Handbook of Behavior Modification and Therapy*. New York: Plenum Press.

Stunkard, A.J., Sorenson, T.I.A., Hanis, C., *et al.* (1986) An adoption study of human obesity. *New England Journal of Medicine*, 314: 193–8.

Sutton, S.R. (1982) Fear-arousing communications: a critical examination of theory and research, in J.R. Eiser (ed.) *Social Psychology and Behavioural Medicine*. Chichester: John Wiley and Sons Ltd.

Sutton, S. (1994) The past predicts the future: Interpreting behaviour-behaviour relationships in social psychological models of health behaviour, in D.R. Rutter and L. Quine (eds) *Social Psychology and Health: European Perspectives*. Aldershot: Avebury.

Sutton, S. (1998) Explaining and predicting intentions and behavior: how well are we doing?, *Journal of Applied Social Psychology*, 28: 1318–39.

Sutton, S.R. (2000) A critical review of the transtheoretical model applied to smoking cessation, in P. Norman, C. Abraham and M. Conner (eds) *Understanding and Changing Health Behaviour: From Health Beliefs to Self-regulation*. Reading: Harwood Academic Press.

Szmukler, G.I. (1989) The psychopathology of eating disorders, in R. Shepherd (ed.) *Handbook of the Physiology of Human Eating*. Chichester: Wiley.

Teff, K.L. and Engelman, K. (1996) Palatability and dietary restraint: effect on cephalic phase insulin release in women, *Physiology and Behavior*, 60: 567–73.

Temple, N.J. (1996) Dietary fats and coronary heart disease, *Biomedicine and Pharmacotherapy*, 50: 261–8.

Temple, N.J. and Walker, A.R.P. (1994) Blood cholesterol and coronary heart disease: changing perspectives, *Journal of the Royal Society of Medicine*, 87: 450.

Thompson, M.M., Zanna, M.P. and Griffin, D.W. (1995) Let's not be indifferent about (attitudinal) ambivalence, in R.E. Petty and J.A. Krosnick (eds) *Attitude Strength: Antecedents and Consequences*. Mahwah, NJ: Lawrence Erlbaum Associates.

Tiggemann, M. (1992) Body-size dissatisfaction: Individual differences in age and gender, and relationship with self-esteem, *Personality and Individual Differences*, 13: 39–43.

Tiggemann, M. and Pennington, B. (1990) The development of gender differences in body-size dissatisfaction, *Australian Psychologist*, 25: 306–13.

Tiggemann, M. and Rothblum, E. (1988) Gender differences and social consequences of perceived overweight in the United States and Australia, *Sex Roles*, 18: 75–86.

Tobin, H. and Logue, A.W. (1994) Self-control across species (columbia-livia, homo-sapiens, and rattus-norvegicus), *Journal of Comparative Psychology*, 108: 126–33.

Toro, J., Cervera, M. and Perez, P. (1988) Body shape, publicity and anorexia nervosa, *Social Psychiatry and Psychiatric Epidemiology*, 23: 132–6.

Towler, G. and Shepherd, R. (1992) Application of Fishbein and Ajzen's expectancy-value model to understanding fat intake, *Appetite*, 18: 15–27.

Triandis, H.C. (1977) *Interpersonal Behavior*. Monterey, CA: Brooks/Cole.

Triplett, N. (1898) The dynamogenic factors in pacemaking and competition, *American Journal of Psychology*, 9: 507–33.

Tuorila, H. (1990) The role of attitudes and preferences in food choice, in J.C. Koskinen (ed.) *Nutritional Adaptation to New Life-styles*. Basel: Karger.

Turk, D.C. and Salovey, P. (1986) Clinical information processing: bias inoculation, in R.E. Ingham (ed.) *Information Processing Approaches to Clinical Psychology*. New York: Academic Press.

Turner, M.R. (1979) *Nutrition and Lifestyles*. London: Elsevier.

van Buerden, E., James, R., Dunn, T. and Tyler, C. (1990) Risk assessment and dietary counselling for cholesterol reduction, *Health Education Research*, 5: 445–50.

van Buskirk, S.S. (1977) A two-phase perspective on the treatment of anorexia nervosa, *Psychological Bulletin*, 84: 529–38.

van den Putte, B. (1991) 20 years of the theory of reasoned action of Fishbein and Ajzen: a meta-analysis. Unpublished manuscript, University of Amsterdam.

van der Pligt, J. and de Vries, N.K. (1998) Belief importance in expectancy-value models of attitudes, *Journal of Applied Social Psychology*, 28: 1339–54.

van der Pligt, J., de Vries, N.K., Manstead, A.S.R. and van Harreveld, F. (2000) The importance of being selective: Weighing the role of attribute importance in attitudinal judgment, *Advances in Experimental Social Psychology*, 32: 135–200.

van Itallie, T.B. (1985) Health implications of overweight and obesity in the United States, *Annals of Internal Medicine*, 103: 983–8.

van Strien, T., Frijters, J.E.R., Bergers, G.P.A. and Defares, P.B. (1986) The Dutch Eating Behaviour Questionnaire for assessment of restrained, emotional and external eating behaviour, *International Journal of Eating Behaviour*, 5: 295–315.

Verbrugge, L.M. (1984) Health diaries – problems and solutions in study design, in C.F. Cannell and R.M. Groves (eds) *Health Survey Research Methods*. DHSS Pub. No. PHS 84–3346. Rockville: National Centre for Health Services Research.

Verplanken, B. and Faes, S. (1999) Good intentions, bad habits, and effects of forming implementation intentions on healthy eating, *European Journal of Social Psychology*, 29: 591–604.

Verplanken, B., Aarts, H. and van Knippenberg, A. (1997) Habit, information acquisition, and the process of making travel mode choices, *European Journal of Social Psychology*, 27: 539–60.

Wardle, J., Steptoe, A., Oliver, G. and Lipsey, Z. (2000) Stress, dietary restraint and food intake, *Journal of Psychosomatic Research*, 48: 195–202.

Warr, P. and Payne, R. (1982) Experiences of strain and pleasure among British adults, *Social Science and Medicine*, 16: 1691–7.

Watson, D. and Hubbard, B. (1996) Adaptational style and dispositional structure: coping in the context of the five factor model, *Journal of Personality*, 64: 737–74.

Weiner, B. (1995) *Judgments of Responsibility: A Foundation for a Theory of Social Conduct*. New York: Guilford Press.

Weinstein, N.D. (1980) Unrealistic optimism about future life events, *Journal of Personality and Social Psychology*, 39: 806–20.

Weinstein, N.D. (1988) The precaution adoption process, *Health Psychology*, 7: 355–86.

Weinstein, N.D., Rothman, A.J. and Sutton, S.R. (1998) Stage theories of health behavior: conceptual and methodological issues, *Health Psychology*, 17: 290–9.

Weinstein, N.D. and Sandman, P.M. (1992) A model of the precaution adoption process: evidence from home radon testing, *Health Psychology*, 11: 170–80.

Weissenberger, J., Rush, A.J., Giles, D.E. and Stunkard, A.J. (1986) Weight change in depression, *Psychiatry Research*, 17: 275–83.

Welty, J.C. (1934) Experiments in group behaviour of fishes, *Physiological Zoology*, 7: 85–128.

Wheeler, L. and Reis, H.T. (1991) Self-recording of everyday life events: origins, types and uses, *Journal of Personality*, 59: 339–54.

White, A., Nicolaas, G., Foster, K., Browne, F. and Carey, S. (1991) *Health survey for England 1991*. London: HMSO.

Wicker, A.W. (1969) Attitudes versus actions: the relationship of verbal and overt behavioral responses to attitude objects, *Journal of Social Issues*, 25: 41–7.

Wilson, T.D., Dunn, D.S., Kraft, D. and Lisle, D.J. (1989) Introspection, attitude change, and attitude–behavior consistency: the disruptive effects of explaining why we feel the way we do, in L. Berkowitz (ed.) *Advances in Experimental Social Psychology*. New York: Academic Press.

Wilson, T.D. and Hodges, S.D. (1992) Attitudes as temporary constructions, in A. Tesser and L. Martin (eds) *The Construction of Social Judgement*. Hillsdale, NJ: Lawrence Erlbaum Associates.

Wilson, T.D., Lindsey, S. and Schooler, T.Y. (2000) A model of dual attitudes, *Psychological Review*, 107: 101–26.

Wing, R.R., Marcus, M.D., Epstein, L.H. and Jawad, A. (1991) A 'family-based' approach to the treatment of obese type II diabetic patients, *Journal of Consulting and Clinical Psychology*, 59: 156–62.

Witte, K. and Allen, M. (2000) A meta-analysis of fear appeals: implications for effective public health campaigns, *Health Education and Behavior*, 27: 591–615.

Wood, P.D., Stefanick, M.L., Williams, P.T. and Haskell, W.L. (1991) The effects on plasma lipoproteins of a prudent weight-reducing diet with or without exercise in overweight men and women, *New England Journal of Medicine*, 325: 461–6.

Woods, S.C., Schwartz, M.W., Baskin, D.G. and Seeley, R.J. (2000) Food intake and the regulation of body weight, *Annual Review of Psychology*, 51: 255–77.

Wurtele, S.K. (1988) Increasing women's calcium intake: the role of health beliefs, intentions, and health value, *Journal of Applied Social Psychology*, 18: 627–39.

Wynder, E.L., Hebert, J.R. and Kabat, G.C. (1987) Association of dietary fat and lung cancer, *Journal of the National Cancer Institute*, 79: 631–7.

Yudkin, J. (1956) Man's choice of food, *The Lancet*, i: 645–9.

Zajonc, R.B. (1965) Social facilitation, *Science*, 149: 269–74.

Zajonc, R.B. (1968) Attitudinal effects of mere exposure, *Journal of Personality and Social Psychology*, 9: 1–27.

Zajonc, R.B., Pietromonaco, P. and Bargh, J.A. (1982) Independence and interaction of affect and cognition, in M.S. Clark and S.T. Fiske (eds) *Affect and Cognition: The Seventeenth Annual Carnegie Symposium on Cognition*. Hillsdale, NJ: Erlbaum.

Zeleznik, W.S. and Bennett, I.M. (1991) Assumption validity in human optimal foraging – the Bari hunters of Venezuela as a test case, *Human Ecology*, 19: 499–508.

Zerbe, K. (1993) *The Body Betrayed: Women, Eating Disorders, and Treatment*. New York: American Psychiatric Press.

Index